An Inquiry Into the Original State and Formation of the Earth; Deduced From Facts and the Laws of Nature. To Which is Added an Appendix, Containing Some General Observations on the Strata in Derbyshire. ... By John Whitehurst

AN INQUIRY

INTO THE

ORIGINAL STATE AND FORMATION

OF THE

EARTH.

A N

INQUIRY

INTO THE

ORIGINAL STATE AND FORMATION

OF THE

EARTH;

DEDUCED FROM FACTS AND THE LAWS OF NATURE.

TO WHICH IS ADDED

AN APPENDIX,

CONTAINING SOME GENERAL OBSERVATIONS ON THE STRATA IN

DERBYSHIRE.

WITH SECTIONS OF THEM, REPRESENTING THEIR ARRANGEMENT, AFFINITIES, AND
THE MUTATIONS THEY HAVE SUFFERED AT DIFFERENT PERIODS OF TIME.
INTENDED TO ILLUSTRATE THE PRECEDING INQUIRIES, AND AS
A SPECIMEN OF SUBTERRANEOUS GEOGRAPHY.

BY JOHN WHITEHURST.

———————————————

LONDON

PRINTED FOR THE AUTHOR, AND W. BENT, BY J. COOPER IN DRURY-
LANE; AND SOLD AT G. ROBINSON's IN PATER-NOSTER ROW.
MDCCLXXVIII.

A

L I S T

OF THE

S U B S C R I B E R S.

A

James Adam, Efq.

Rev. Mr. Adams, rector of South-ockington, Effex.

Stanefby Alchorne, Efq. Affay-mafter to the Mint.

Thomas Allen, Efq.

Mr. Arnold, watchmaker.

—— Afhton, Efq. Liverpool.

Mr. Atkinfon, Congleton, Che-fhire, *four books.*

Geo. Atwood, Efq. M. A. F. R. S. fellow of Trin. Coll. Camb.

Alexander Aubert, Efq. F. R. S. *two books.*

John Aufrere, Efq. Chelfea.

Wm. Auftin, Efq. M. A. Wad-ham College, Oxford.

John Ayre, jun. Efq. Tilton, Lei-cefterfhire.

B

The Right Hon. the Earl of Bef-borough.

Sir Robert Burdett, Bart. Fore-mark, Derbyfhire.

Sir Robert Barker, Bart.

Sir George Beaumont, Bart.

Sir William Bagot, Bart.

Mr. Baddely, Surgeon, Newport, Shropfhire.

Mr. Robert Bage, Elford, Staf-fordfhire.

Mr. Charles Bage, land-furveyor, Salop.

Robert Bakewell, Efq. Greffley, Derbyfhire.

Mr. Charles Baker, London.

John Balguy, Efq. Alfreton, Der-byfhire.

Mr. Samuel Ball, Tamworth, Warwickfhire.

Jofeph Banks, Efq. F. R. S. Soho-Square.

Alexander Barker, Efq. Edenfor, Derbyfhire.

Mr. John Barker, ditto.

Mr. George Barker, ditto.

Mr. Alexander Barker, ditto.

John Barker, Efq. Bakewell, Der-byfhire.

The Rev. Mr. Barker, Youl-grave, ditto.

Samuel

LIST OF SUBSCRIBERS.

Samuel Barlow, Efq. Maleverer, Yorkfhire.

Mr. Charles Barnes, Cheadle, Staffordfhire.

Mr. Thomas Baines, Plumber, Chefter.

John Barratt, Efq.

Francis Baffet, Efq. St Minver, Cornwall.

Mifs Bateman, Derby.

—— Bates, M. D. Miffenden, Bucks, *two books*.

John Bawdler, Efq. Inner-Temple.

Rowland Bayley, Efq.

Richard Beauvoir, Efq.

Rev. Mr. Becher, prebendary of Southwell.

John Beech, Efq Shaw, Staffordfhire.

Richard Benyon, Efq. *two books*.

Mr. Bent, Surgeon, Newcaftle, Staffordfhire.

Thomas Bentley, Efq. Turnham-Green, *four books*.

John Berridge, M. D. Derby.

Rev. Charles Berridge, LL.D. Cambridge.

Francis Beiresford, Efq. Afhburn, Derbyfhire.

Peregrine Bertie, Efq.

Rev Mr. Bill, Draycott, Staffordfhire.

Mr. Bilfborrow, attorney, Derby.

Thomas Birch, Efq.

George Birch, Efq.

Mr. Bland, Surgeon, Newark, Nottinghamfhire.

Mr. John Booth, Sheffield.

Mr. John Boultbee.

Mr. Thomas Boultbee.

Matthew Boulton, Efq. Soho, Staffordfhire.

Mr. Bradley, jun. Birchover, Derbyfhire.

Frederick Browning, Efq. fellow of King's Coll. Cambridge.

Mr. James Brock, Buxton, Derbyfhire.

Mr. Job Charlton Brough, Newark, Nottinghamfhire, *two books*

Mr. Ifaac Brown, London.

Mrs. Brown, Norfolk.

Jacob Bryant, Efq.

William Bullock, M. D. Afhford, Derbyfhire.

Rev. Mr. John Bullock.

Mrs. Burn, Olderfhaw, Staffordfhire.

Rev. Mr. Burflem, fellow of St. John's Coll. Cambridge.

Mr. Buxton, furgeon, Buxton, Derbyfhire.

Mr. Edward Buxton, furgeon, Bakewell, Derbyfhire.

C

The Right Hon. Lord Clive.

The Right Hon. Lord Geo. Cavendifh, *two books*.

The Right Hon. Lord Fred. Cavendifh.

The Right Hon. Lord John Pelham Clinton.

The Hon. Lord Compton, Trin. Coll. Cambridge.

The Hon. Henry Cavendifh. F. R. S.

The Hon Henry Cecil, Hanbury, Worcefterfhire.

LIST OF SUBSCRIBERS.

Sir James Clerk, Bart. Penny-cuick, Scotland, *two books.*

The Hon. Francis Cuft, Efq. Lincoln's Inn.

Mr. Chriftopher Carpenter.

John Carr, Efq. York.

George Carter, Efq. Margaret-Street, Cavendifh-Square.

Mr. Henry Cartwright, Coal-Moor

Henry Boult Cay, Efq.

Geo. Chamberlayne, Efq. King's Coll. Cambridge.

William Chamberlayne, Efq. folicitor to the Treafury

Chriftopher Chambers, Efq. London.

Thomas Charlton, Efq. Trinity Coll. Cambridge.

Mr. Charlton.

Mr John Chatterton, plumber, Derby.

Robert Cheney, Efq. Meynell Langley, Derbyfhire.

Rev Mr Chapman, Bakewell, Derbyfhire.

Mr Clark, plaifterer, Weftminfter.

Rev. Mr. Clarkfon, Derby.

Rev Mr. James Clay, Rofeby-Broom, Yorkfhire.

Mr. William Clay, Wefthorpe, Nottinghamfhire.

Dan. Parker Coke, Efq. Derby.

Mr. Collins, carpenter, Greenwich.

Rev. William Cooper, D. D. prebendary of Southwell.

Mr. William Cooper, furgeon, Salop.

Mr. Jof. Cooper, printer, London.

Thomas Copley, Efq. Doncafter.

John Corbet, Efq. Sundorn, Salop.

Thomas Cotton, Efq.

Kenton Coufe, Efq. Scotland-yard.

Mr. George Creffwell, Afhford, Derbyfhire.

John Crewe, Efq. Bolefworth-Caftle, Chefhire.

Mr. Thomas Crichlow, Liverpool Infirmary.

John Cuthbert, Efq. F. R. S. Inner-Temple.

D

Mr. Emanuel Mendes Da Cofta.

Mr Michael Daintry, Leek, Staffordfhire

Mr. John Daintry, ditto.

Mr. Dakin, plumber, Berner's Street.

Alexander Dalrymple, Efq.

Mr. Darby, Colebrook-Dale, *two books.*

Robert. Darwin, Efq. Elfton, Nottinghamfhire.

Erafmus Darwin, M. D. F. R. S. Litchfield.

Charles Vere Dafhwood, Efq. of Stanford, Leicefterfhire.

D. C. Davenport, Efq. Wellerton.

Mr. John Davenport, Ball-Hay, Staffordfhire, *two books.*

Mr. Henry Davenport, mafon, Leek, Staffordfhire.

Thomas Day, Efq.

Mrs. Delany, St. James's Place.

Mr. Denby, organift, Derby.

——— Den-

LIST OF SUBSCRIBERS.

—— Denman, M. D. Bakewell, Derbyshire.

Rev. Mr. John Derby, M. A. chaplain to the Bishop of Rochester, and rector of Southfleet and Longfield in Kent.

Mr. William Defanges.

Mr. Deval, mason.

John Dewes, Esq.

Bernard Dewes, Esq.

Rev. Mr Dickenson, Blimmil,

Thomas Dickins, Esq Drayton, Salop.

Mr. Dickinson of Taxal.

Rev. Dr. Disney, Flentham, Nottingham.

Matthew Dobson, M. D. Liverpool

Mr. Dobbinson, Derby.

Rev. Dr. Douglas.

William Drake, Esq. Amersham, Bucks.

William Drake, jun Esq. ditto.

Matthew Duane, Esq. F. R. S.

Jeremiah Dyson, Esq.

E

The Right Hon. the Earl of Exeter.

Geo. Edwards, M. D Wigmore-Street, Cavendish-Square.

Rev. Mr John Edwards.

Philip Egerton, Esq Oulton, Cheshire, *six books.*

Mr. John Eginton, Soho, Staffordshire.

Mr. Francis Eginton, ditto.

Mr. Emes, gardener, Bowbridge-field, Derbyshire, *four books.*

Thomas Emlyn, Esq. F. R. S. John-Street, Gray's-Inn.

Rev. Mr. Empsom, A. B. Catherine-Hall, Cambridge.

Rev. Dr. Enfield, Warrington.

Rev. Mr English, chaplain to the 25th regiment.

Mr. English, hosier, Cheapside.

Mr. Benjamin Eyre, Tokenhouse-Yard.

Thomas Eyre, Esq. Hassop, Derbyshire.

F

The Right Hon. Earl Ferrers.

The Hon. Thomas Fitzmaurice.

Mr. James Ferguson, Academy in Hermitage-Street.

Rev. Charles Fienes, Newark, Nottinghamshire.

Mr Fletcher, land-surveyor, Heynel, Derbyshire.

Mr. John Flint, Salop.

Mr. Cornelius Flint, Great Longston, Derbyshire.

Mr. Flint.

Mr. Fox, surgeon, Leicester.

Mr. Ingham Foster, Clement's-Lane.

Richard French, Esq. *two books.*

Mr. French, attorney, Uppingham, Rutland.

G

The Right Hon. Lord Viscount Gage.

Mr.

LIST OF SUBSCRIBERS.

Sir Sampſon Gideon, Bart.

The Hon Charles Greville, F R S.

Philip Gell, Eſq. Hopton, Derbyſhire.

Capt. Gell, No. 20, Orchard-
Street.

Mr. Getcliff, ſurgeon, Cheadle,
Staffordſhire.

Mr James Gibbons Light-Moor.

Rev. Mr Giffard, rector of Nor-
thockington, Eſſex

Thomas Gilbert Eſq Cotton, Staffordſhire

Mr. John Gilbert, Worſley, Lan-
caſhire.

William Maun, Godſchall, Eſq.

The Rev. Mr Godwin, Gataker.

George Goodman, Eſq. Tixal,
Derbyſhire.

Mr. William Goodwin.

Mr. William Greaves, plumber,
Bakewell, Derbyſhire.

Mr Green, Walworth, Surry.

Mr. Green, ſurgeon, Litchfield.

Rev. Dr. Greſley, Nether Seal,
Derbyſhire

Rev. Mr Gretton, rector of Norton, Salop

Rev. Mr Gretton, A. B. Trin.
Coll. Cambridge

Mr. Thomas Griffin, Longſton,
Staffordſhire.

Ralph Griffith, Eſq. Turnham-
Green.

Mr. Groves, ſen. Weſtminſter.

Mr. Groves, jun. ditto.

Mr. Bartlet Gurney, Norwich,
two books.

— Guthrie, M. D. St. Peterſburgh.

H

The Right Hon. the Earl of Hard-
wicke.

The Right Hon. Sir Wm Hamilton, K B. his Majeſty's plenipotentiary at Naples.

The Hon Mrs. How.

The Hon. Arthur Holdſworth,
governor of Dartmouth Caſtle.

Sir Thomas Heathcote, Bart.

Mr Haggit, B. A Trinity Coll.
Cambridge.

Mr William Haigh, Tideſwell,
Derbyſhire.

Mr John Halifax, ſurgeon, Newcaſtle, Nottinghamſhire.

Mr Michael Hall, attorney, Ca-
ſtleton, Derbyſhire.

Mr. Richard Harper, Shrewſbury.

Mr. Harrison, watchmaker, Liverpool.

Mr. William Heaford, Eccleſhall,
Staffordſhire.

Samuel Heathcote Eſq. Littleover,

William Heberden, M. D. and
F. R. S.

Mr Hen Hegg, druggiſt, Cheſter.

The Rev. Mr. Hemmington.

Lieut. Logan Henderſon, of the
marines

Stanhope Hervey, Eſq. Womer-
ſley, Yorkſhire

John Hewet, Eſq. Shire-Oakes,
Nottinghamſhire, *two books.*

Mr. Richard Hill, Farley, Staffordſhire.

Mr. William Hodges, landſcape-
painter.

b   Mr.

LIST OF SUBSCRIBERS.

Mr Hodgkinson, attorney. Southwell, Nottinghamshire

—— Hodgson, Esq Coleman-Street

Robert Hodgson, Esq Congleton, Cheshire.

Mr Hodgson, distiller, Stratford.

Mr B Hodgson, Buxton, Derbyshire

Robert Holden, Esq Darley, ditto.

Atkinson Holden, Esq ditto

T. Holles, Esq Great Ormond-Street.

Mr Holmes, Wandsworth.

John Barker Holroyd, Esq. Sheffield-Place, Sussex

Mr John Holt, Walton, Lancashire

Rev Mr. Hope, Derby.

Joseph Hornby, Esq. Gainsborough

Mr George Horsington, Chelsea College.

The Rev. Dr. Horsley, F. R. S.

Mr Robert How, Castleton, Derbyshire

—— Howard, Esq Sheffield.

Richard Hulse, Esq.

John Hunter, M.D. F R.S. Leicester-Fields, *two books.*

The Rev. Mr Hurst, Stanford, Leicestershire.

Mr. Rob Hyman, watchmaker to her Imperial Maj. of Russia.

I

Sir Richard Jebb, Bart. M. D.

Richard Jackson, Esq.

—— Jackson, M. D. Stamford, Lincolnshire.

Rev Mr. Jay, Smeaton, Yorkshire.

John Ibbetson, Esq. F. R. S. Greenwich.

Henry Jervise, Esq.

Mr Ince, attorney, Wirksworth, Derbyshire.

Mr Joseph Ingleby, Cheadle, Staffordshire

William Johnson, Esq. M. A. King's College, Cambridge.

Rev. Mr. Jones.

Mr Jones, bookseller, Wrexam.

Rev. Mr. Wm. Judgson, Bolesworth-Castle, Cheshire.

Mr. Jupp.

K

James Keir, Esq.

John Kenrick, Esq. commissioner of stamps

King's Coll. Library, Cambridge.

—— Kirkland, M. D. Ashby de la Zouch, Leicestershire.

Mr. Kyte, surgeon, Gravesend.

Mr. Edward Kynaston, St. John's College, Cambridge.

L

The Right Hon. Lord Lisburne.

The Right Hon. Lord Le Despenser.

The Right Hon. the Earl of Lincoln.

The Right Hon. the Countess of Lincoln.

Sir

LIST OF SUBSCRIBERS.

Sir Afhton Lever, Leicefter-Fields.

Mr. Latham, furgeon, Bromley, Kent.

Rev. Mr. Law, Southwell, Nottinghamfhire.

Charlwood Lawton, Efq.

Anthony Lax, Efq. Chefterfield, Derbyfhire.

Edward Leacroft, Efq Langley, Derbyfhire.

Mr John Leacroft, attorney, Wirkfworth, dito.

Mr Wm Leatham, Bafinghall-Street, *four books*

Mr. Bofwell Leatham, ditto, *three books.*

Edward Leigh, Efq Green-Hill, Staffordfhire, *three books.*

Francis Leigh, Efq.

Henry Cornwall Leigh, Efq.

Mr. Rupert Leigh.

Mr. Francis Leigh.

Mr. John Leonard, Alderfhaw, Staffordfhire.

Mr. Leverts.

C. Rand Lewis, Efq. Suffex.

Mr Lewis.

Liverpool Library.

Rev. Mr. Lindfay, M. A.

Rev. Mr. Lock, Newark, Nottinghamfhire.

William Longfton, Efq. Eyam, Derbyfhire

Mr. James Longfton, Longfton, Derbyfhire.

William Lowther, Efq. Trinity College, Cambridge

John Loyd, Efq. F R S Temple 2 *books.*

Edward Lucas, Efq Lambeth.

Jof Lucas, Efq affay-mafter, Mint.

Rev. William Ludlam, M. A. Leicefter.

M

The Right Hon. Lord Mulgrave.

—— Maddox, Efq. Temple.

Mr. Mander, attorney, Bakewell, Derbyfhire.

Mr. Samuel Mander, attorney, Temple.

Mr Manley, attorney, Chefterfield.

Colonel Mafter, Hull.

Tho. March, Efq Bedford Row.

—— Marfden, Efq fellow commoner, Trin Coll. Cambridge.

Rev. Dr. Mafkyline, Aftronomer Royal and F. R. S.

Mr. Mafon, Matlock.

Mr. John Marfon, Clumber-Houfe, Nottinghamfhire.

Mr. Mathewman, Sheffield.

Mr. William Mathews, merchant, London.

Rev Mr Mellequet, Little Budworth, Chefhire.

Wm Mellifh, Efq. receiver-general.

Charles Mellifh, Efq.

Jofeph Mellifh, Efq

Mr. Jof. Mellor, Leek, Staffordfhire

Mr Wm Mettam, Eyam, Derbyfhire.

Rev Mr. Middleton

—— Miller, M. D London.

Rev Mr. Milnes, Newark, Nottinghamfhire

Rev Mr. Mills, Derbyfhire

Mr. Moor, fecretary to the Society of Arts and Commerce.

Charles

LIST OF SUBSCRIBERS.

Charles Morton, M. D. F. R. S. and principal librarian to the British Muſeum.

Richard Motard, Eſq.

Mr. John Bailey Madeley, ſurgeon, Uttoxeter, Staffordſhire.

Mr. Murrev, Burleigh.

Mrs Myddleton, Amerſham, Buckinghamſhire.

Richard Mydleton, Eſq.

N

His Grace the Duke of Newcaſtle, *five books.*

The Rt. Hon. Sir Fletcher Norton, Speaker of the Houſe of Commons.

Mrs. Nicolls, Swithamley.

Peter Nightingale, Eſq Lee, Derbyſhire

L. Norcup, Eſq. Tunſtal, Shropſhire.

O

—— Oakes, M. D Mansfield, Nottinghamſhire.

Walter Oburn, Eſq. Ravensfield, Yorkſhire.

Peter Oliver, Eſq Maſſachuſets-Bay.

Thomas Ottley, Eſq Pitchford.

Rev Mr Outlaw, Northamptonſhire.

P

The Right Hon. the Earl of Powis.

Sir John Pringle, Bart. preſident of the Royal Society.

John Paradice, Eſq.

Mr. James Parke, Liverpool.

Edward Parker, Eſq. Brigg.

George Parker, Eſq. Amington, Salop.

Mr. Parkinſon, Newport, ditto.

Rev. Mr. Paſhley, Barlborough, Derbyſhire.

James Payne, Eſq.

Rev. Mr. Peach, Derby.

John Peachy, Eſq.

Charles Anderſon Pelham, Eſq. Brocklesby, Lincolnſhire, *ſix books.*

Mr George Pengree, Sheffield.

Mr. William Pengree, ditto.

Mr. Perchard, ſurgeon.

—— Percival, M. D. Mancheſter.

George Perry, Eſq Weſtminſter.

Mr. John Philips, Fean, Staffordſhire.

Mr Nathaniel Philips, Mancheſter.

Mr. John Philips, Mancheſter.

Mr. N Philips, Mancheſter.

Colonel Philipſon.

Rev Mr. Pickering, Mackworth, Derbyſhire, *two books.*

Rev. Mr. William Pickering, ditto.

Charles Pigott, Eſq Peplow.

Thomas Pigott, Eſq.

Mr. John Platts, Rotherham.

Roger Pocklington, Eſq. Winthorpe.

Mr. Robert Pointer.

Rev. Dr Pollock

Edward Poore, Eſq

John Port, Eſq. Ilam, Staffordſhire.

Rev. Mr. Porter, M A. fellow of Trinity Coll Cambridge.

Rev.

LIST OF SUBSCRIBERS.

Rev. Mr. Prefton.
Rev. Dr. Price.
Rev. Dr. Prieftly.
John Probert, Efq. Shropfhire.
Rev. Mr. Prior, Afhby de la Zouch, Leiceft-rfhire.
Dan. Pulteney, Efq. M. A. King's Coll. Cambridge.

R

The Right Hon. the Marquis of Rockingham.
The Right Hon Lord Ravenf-worth.
Sir John Rufhout, Bart.
Rev. Mr. Raikes, Neufden, *two books.*
Matthew Raper, Efq. F. R. S. *two books.*
Rev. Dr. Raftal, Prebendary of Southwell.
Rev. S. Raftal, Newark.
Mr. T. Rawfon, Nottingham.
Mr. Rehe, Shoe-Lane, London.
Mr. Rennard, fugar-baker, Hull.
Mr. John Reynolds, Plafto, Der-byfhire.
Mr. Reynolds, Ketley.
Mr. William Reynolds.
Richard Reynolds, Efq. Raxton, Huntingdonfhire.
Mr. Reynolds, Kettlebank.
John Rhodes, Efq. Balborough, Derbyfhire, *two books.*
Anthony Rhudde, Efq.
Dr. Rogerfon, phyfician to the Emprefs of Rufha.
Lancelot Rolleston, Efq. Watnall, Nottinghamfhire.

—— Ripley, Efq.
Rev. John Edward Rollefton.
Mr. Rofe, plaifterer.
William Ruffel, Efq. F. R. S. *four books.*

S

The Right Hon. the Earl of Shel-burne.
The Right Hon. the Earl of Sea-forth.
The Right Hon. Lord Scarfdale, *two books.*
The Right Hon. Lady Scarfdale.
Sir George Savile, Bart. *two books.*
Sir George Shuckburgh, Bart.
Mr. Sale, woollen-draper, Derby.
Mr. John Salt, Wirkfworth, Der-byfhire.
Rev. Mr. Sandys, rector of St. Minver, Cornwall.
John Sargent, Efq. Halfted, Kent.
George Sargent, Arnold Efq.
John Sargent Efq jun,
Mr. Scott.
Robert Shuttleworth, Efq.
Jofeph Sikes, Efq. Newark.
Mr. Shakefpear.
Rev Mr. Shaw, rector of Smeaton, Yorkfhire.
Mr. Shore, Snitterton, Derbyfhire.
Mr. Slaughter, Longford, Shrop-fhire
Mr Smedley, Youlgreave, Der-byfhire.
John Sneyd, Efq. Belmont, Staf-fordfhire.
Mr. Snowden, Clement's Inn.
Dr. Solander, F. R S.

South-

Southwell Book-Society.
Mr Thomas Sparrow.
—— Spence, M D Derby.
Mr Thomas Stamford, Derby.
George Stewart, Esq.
James Stuart, Esq F. R. S.

T

Mr. Anthony Tiffington, Alfreton, Derbyshire.
Miss Tiffington, Winster, ditto.
Henry Tolcher, sen. Esq. Plymouth.
Mr. Touchett, Manchester.
Mr George Townshend.
Mr Richard Trevis, Chatsworth.
Trinity College, Cambridge.
Mr. Henry Tudor, Sheffield.
Mr. Matthew Turner, surgeon, Liverpool.
Mr. Samuel Turner, Attorney, Nottingham, *two books.*
Rev. Mr. Turner.
James Twigg, Esq A. B. St. John's College, Cambridge.
Mr John Twigg, Bakewell.
F. John Tyssen, Esq.

V

Mr. Benjamin Vaughan, Mincing-Lane.
Mr. William Vaughan, ditto.

W

Rev. Mr. Wade, A. B. St. John's College, Cambridge.
Dr. John Wadsworth, Sheffield.

Mr. Ezekiel Walker, Lynn.
Dr. Walker, Hull, Yorkshire.
Mr. Wall
Edward Waller, Esq Beaconsfield.
John Walsh, Esq. F. R. S. *two books.*
Mr. Walton, Repton, Derbyshire.
Rev Mr Ward.
Rev. John Ward.
Richard Hill Waring, Esq. Leeswood, Flintshire.
Samuel Watson, Esq. Hull, Yorkshire.
Mr. Thomas Watson, Sheffield.
Mr. Henry Watson, Bakewell, Derbyshire.
Jos. Wedgwood, Esq *two books.*
Samuel Wegg, Esq
Mr. Weston, enameller, Quaker's Buildings, West Smithfield.
Mr Westwood.
William Wheat, Esq. Sheffield, *two books.*
Martin Whish, Esq. commissioner of stamps, *four books.*
Mr. White, Westminster.
Snowden White, M. D. Nottingham, *two books.*
Capt. Rich. Wilding, Liverpool
Rev. Mr. Wilding, Prescott Lane.
Mr. Wilkinson, apothecary, Liverpool Infirmary.
Mr. Wilkinson, Oulton.
John Wilkinson, Esq. Brofeley.
Joseph Williams. Esq. Carnarvonshire.
Rev. Mr. Williams, *three books.*
Mr. William Wale, Master of the Mathematical School, Christ's Hospital.

—— Wills,

LIST OF SUBSCRIBERS.

—— Wills, Efq. New-Inn.
Mr. Robert Wilmot, plaifterer.
Mr. Winchefter, Bakewell, Der-
byfhire.
Mr. Winter, Manchefter.
Hans Winthorpe, Mortimer, Efq.
Samuel Pipe Wolverfton, Efq.
near Tamworth.

Mr. Thomas Woodhoufe, Crich,
Derbyfhire.
Stephen Wright, Efq. Scotland-
Yard, *two books*.
—— Wright, M. D. Newark.
Mr. Wylde, Mansfield.
Ifaac Lafcels Wynn, Efq. Jamaica.

OMITTED.

Rev. William Chambers, D. D. Derby.
Rev. Mr. Michell, M. A. F. R. S.
Mr. E. R. Rafpe.
Rev. Mr. Rivett, M. A.
Mr. Ifaac Swainfon.
Mr. Young, furgeon, Fenchurch-ftreet, London.
Mr. Young, furgeon, Sheffnal, Shropfhire.

ERRATA.

Page 14, l. 1, for *instantaneous*, read *instantaneously*.
    33, l. 10, from the bottom, for *echenites*, r. *echinites*.
    34, l. 8, and p 37, l. 3, from the bottom, for *glossopetra*, r. *glossopetræ*.
    51, l. 22, for *gaden*, r *garden*.
    59, l 7, and p 79, l 24, for 1538, r 1638.
    70, l 6, for *Borelleus*, r. *Borellus*.
    94, l. 6, for *tha*, r *that* , l 8, from the bottom, after *than* r *the*.
    128, l 12, for *on*, r. *of*.
    137, l 20, and p 138, l. 10, for *Varanius*, r. *Varenius*.
    160. l. 7, plate ix. fig 2, refers to a *plan* and not a *section*.
    163, l. 5, from the bottom, for *lava*, r. *toadstone*.
    192, l 11, for *the* r *their*.
The *omission* of the *tenth chapter* is only an error of the press.

PREFACE.

AFTER fo many volumes have been written to inveftigate the original ftate and formation of the earth,
and the changes it has undergone, it may appear
prefumptuous to offer my fentiments to the public
on fo extenfive a fubject.

But when it is confidered, that the book of Nature
is open to all men, and perhaps in no part of the world
more fo than in Derbyfhire, the wonder will ceafe ;
for natural phenomena fo plentifully abound, that pa-
tience and affiduity are only needful to examine thofe
things which have a tendency to unfold the original
ftate and formation of the earth, and the changes it
has undergone. It may appear wonderful, that amidft
all the confufion of the *ftrata*, there is neverthelefs
one conftant invariable order in the arrangement of
them, and their various productions of animal, vegetable, and mineral fubftances, or rather the figures or impreffions of the two former. Thefe appearances engaged my attention very early in life, to fearch and inquire into the various caufes of them, and I hope that
the facts which I have afcertained from my own ob-

A   fervation,

fervation, and collected from feveral experienced mineis, if not the inferences deduced fiom them, will entitle the following pages to a candid examination.

This woik is not wholly calculated for the enteitainment of fpeculative minds; but, in part, to eftablifh fuch a fyftem of Subteiraneous Geography, as may in time become fubfeivient to the purpofes of human life, by leading to the difcoveiy of thofe things which are concealed from our obfervation in the lower regions of the earth.

The feveral theories already pioduced contain, indeed, many impoitant truths; yet it muft be owned, that, in fome inftances, they are too hypothetical for an age which only admits of deductions from FACTS, and the LAWS of NATURE. It has not, however, been the object of my attention to point out the faults of other fyftems; but to avail myfelf of fuch parts of them as were applicable to my own defign, to DERIVE the NATURE OF THINGS from CAUSES TRULY EXISTENT, and to INQUIRE after thofe LAWS by which the CREATOR CHOSE to FORM THE WORLD; and not THOSE on which HE MIGHT have FORMED IT, had HE fo pleafed.

CONTENTS.

CONTENTS.

C H A P.

CONTENTS.

AN

AN

INQUIRY

INTO THE

ORIGINAL STATE AND FORMATION

OF THE

EARTH.

CHAP. I.

Introduction. Of the Laws of Gravity, Fluidity, and Centrifugal Force. Of the original State of the Earth; of its diurnal Rotation; Beginning; and the Mode of its first Existence.

THE number of ages elapsed, since the DEITY created the constituent parts of the earth, and assembled them together by the law of universal gravitation, will not, I presume, admit of a philosophical investigation, whilst natural phenomena remain in so much obscurity; therefore, the chronological history of the earth cannot be truly ascertained from physical *data*, nor

B   any

any lights borrowed from its great antiquity to found thefe reafonings upon.   Hence we are obliged to leave the decifion of that important matter, until further dif-coveries are made ; and, for the prefent, confine our refearches to unfold the original ftate and formation of the earth, and the changes it has undergone.

Sir Ifaac Newton hath happily laid the foundation for a natural hiftory of the terraqueous globe, by de-monftrating its figure to be an oblate fpheroid-----that its equatorial diameter exceeds its polar diameter upwards of thirty-four miles, or in the ratio of 230 to 229.   Upon this fingle truth, and its coincidence with the laws of gravity, fluidity and centrifugal force, the following Inquiry muft ftand or fall , for although the facts are innumerable which ferve to illuftrate the ori-ginal ftate of the earth ; yet its oblate fpheroidical form may truly be confidered as the only natural *da-tum* on which the fubject can be eftablifhed, and the only teft by which its truth can be examined.

Previous to that great difcovery, every one thought himfelf at liberty to model the earth according to the dictates of his own fancy ; whence arofe various con-jectures concerning its magnitude and figure, to the great embarraffment of aftronomy, geography, and na-vigation : and although the refult of Sir Ifaac's reafon-

ings

ings were deduced from the unerring laws of Nature, yet his demonstration was not immediately received, and therefore only served to increase the general confusion of preceding opinions, for several years after his decease.

However, to the immortal honour of the French nation, the Royal Academy of Sciences represented to their Sovereign the necessity of determining the magnitude and figure of the earth by the actual mensuration of a degree of the meridian near the equator, and likewise in the polar regions, in order to ascertain their curvatures, and from their equalities or inequalities to deduce its true figure and magnitude.

This princely and hazardous enterprize was undertaken in Lapland, by command of Lewis XV. and executed in the years 1736 and 1737, by Messis. Maupertuis, Camus, Clairaut, and Le Monier, members of the Royal Academy of Sciences : and in a few years after, the equatorial observations were completed, by command of the King of Spain, by Don George Juan, Don Antonia Ulloa, M. Condamine, &c. The result was as follows :

The equatorial diameter $= 7940,598$
The polar diameter $= 7903,650$
English miles.

Hence

Hence it appears that the equatorial diameter exceeds the polar 36₁₈₈₈ miles ; which fo nearly coincides with Sir Ifaac's theoretical demonftration, that the magnitude and figure of the earth were determined with fufficient accuracy, to the great joy of the philofophic world, the improvement of fcience, and of natural hiftory.

Mr. Graham, our celebrated countryman, was principally concerned in conftructing the apparatus for-furveying the polar regions.

Now fince the figure of the earth and the laws of motion are confidered as the principal *data*, whence the following refearches are derived, I hope my learned readers will allow me to premife fome neceffary propofitions, to render the fubfequent reafonings more familiar to thofe who have not been converfant with fuch fpeculations ; for without fome previous knowledge of the principles whence the earth acquired its oblate fpheroidical form, it will be altogether in vain to proceed one ftep farther.

PROPOSITION I.

According to the univerfal law of gravitation, the conftituent parts of all bodies mutually attract each other : hence arifes a common center of gravity, which fo governs their component parts, as to caufe all fuch as are *fluid* and at *reft*, to affume fpherical forms.

For example. If two equal particles of matter mutually attract each other at any given diftance, as at A and B, fig. I. they will move towards

Fig I.

A · · · C · · B

each other, with equal velocities, in the direction A C and B C, and confequently will come into contact at the mean diftance C ; therefore the point C may be confidered as their common center of gravity.

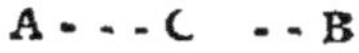

Again : If three particles of matter mutually attract each other at A B C, fig. II. they will alfo move with equal velocities towards each other, in the direction A D, B D, C D ; and therefoie will come into contact in the point D : confequently, the point D becomes their common center of gravity.

A　*Fig.* II.

·D·

c · · · B

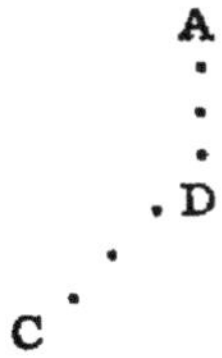

If four particles of matter mutually attract each other at A B C D, fig. III. they will alfo move towards each other in the directions A E, B E, C E, D E ; therefore the point E may be confidered as their center of gravity.

A　*Fig.* III.

D · · · E · · · B

C

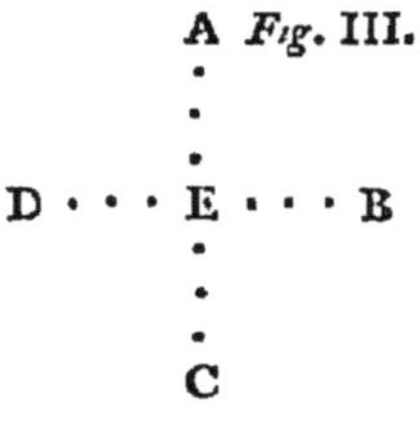

This

This law is well known to hold univerfally true, whatever be the number of particles thus attracted ; whence it follows, that the center of gravity in all bodies arifes from the law of mutual attraction ; and therefore when the component parts of fluid bodies are thus affembled together, they muft neceffarily affume fpherical forms, to reftore the equilibrium of gravitation : as drops of water, mercury, or melted metal.

Now fince there are no other laws or principles in nature yet known, whence bodies can affume fpherical forms, but thofe of *gravity, fluidity* and *reft,** it feems reafonable to conclude, that all bodies naturally fpherical muft have been originally in a ftate of *fluidity* and *reft,* though they may be *firm* and *folid* in their prefent ftate.

PROPOSITION II.

According to the univerfal laws of motion, the conftituent parts of all bodies which revolve upon their axes acquire a centrifugal force, in proportion to their velocities : therefore, as their diftances are to each other from their axes of motion, fo are their velocities, and fo are their centrifugal forces.

* By bodies at *reft* is here meant fuch as do not revolve upon their axes.

For

For example: Let fig. 1. plate V. reprefent an equatorial fection of a globe, or the plane of its equator; and let us fuppofe its radius divided into fix equal parts, by the concentric circles 1, 2, 3, 4, 5, 6; and let us again fuppofe that it revolves upon its axis A with any given velocity : hence it follows, by induction, that the velocity of the particles contained in each circle will increafe, according to their refpective diftances from their axis of motion A : and therefore, as their velocities are to each other, fo are their centrifugal forces.

Again : Let fig. 2, plate V. reprefent the polar fection of a globe, A A its axis, and E E its equator; and let us fuppofe its radius divided into fix equal parts, by the lines 1, 2, 3, 4, 5, 6, running parallel to the axis A A : hence it will follow, according to the former diagram, that the velocity and centrifugal force of the particles contained in each line will increafe according to their refpective diftances from their axis of motion A A.

Now as the centrifugal force in the axis A A is nothing, and gradually increafes from C to E E; it evidently follows, that the equilibrium of gravitation is deftroyed in all revolving bodies; and therefore fuch as revolve upon their axes in a ftate of fluidity will

depart

depart from a fpherical form, and affume that of an oblate fpheroid, whofe equatorial diameters will exceed their polar diameters in a certain ratio, according to their periodical rotations.

Such are the confequences arifing from the unalterable laws of gravity, fluidity, and centrifugal force ; and therefore fince there are no other laws or principles in nature yet known, whence bodies can acquire oblate fpheroidical forms, it evidently follows, that all oblate fpheroidical bodies have turned round their axes in a ftate of fluidity, although they may be *firm* and *folid* in their prefent ftate.

Therefore, fince the figure of the earth has been demonftrated to be an oblate fpheroid----and likewife, that its equatorial diameter exceeds its polar, in proportion to the velocity of its diurnal rotation ; it neceffarily follows, that its oblate fpheroidical form *muft* have been acquired by *revolving* on its axis in a ftate of FLUIDITY.

Now fince it appears, that the figure of the earth fo perfectly coincides with the laws of motion, may we not conclude, that its diurnal rotation has fuffered no *change* or *variation* ; but, according to the immutable laws of Nature, it has performed equal rotations in equal times, throughout all ages of the world.

Having

Having thus confidered the original ftate of this great globle, and the equality of its days, from the creation to the prefent time ; it becomes neceffary to inquire whether its fluidity was owing to any diffolvent principle, or to the firft affemblage of its component parts.

It will be readily granted, that the earth was brought into exiftence either in a folid or in a fluid ftate---If the former, it muft have been *diffolved*, and this by fome univerfal *diffolvent principle* : therefore, as no fuch principle is yet known to exift in nature, is it not reafonable to conclude, that its fluidity was owing to the *firft affemblage* of its component parts, and not to any fubfequent folution ? Hence it appears, that the earth had a beginning, and cannot have exifted from eternity, as fome perfons have imagined.

C CHAP.

CHAP. II.

Of the Chaotic State of the Earth.

TAKING for granted that the globe which we now inhabit was originally in a ftate of fluidity, let us endeavour to afceitain the confequences neceffarily arifing from that particular ftate and condition of it.

The fluidity of the earth evidently fhews, that the particles of matter which now compofe the *ftrata*, and all othei folid bodies, were not originally united, combined, oi fixed by cohefion, but actually in a ftate of feparation, like the particles of fugar or falt fufpended in water.

Now it is a truth univerfally known, that the component parts of the moft denfe bodies become fufpended, in whatever *menftrua* they are diffolved : as gold in *aqua regia*, filver in *aqua fortis*, falts in *water*, and water in *air* : nay, even mercury, in the act of diftillation, becomes fufpended in aii, although the fpecific gravity of the foimei is, at leaft, eleven thoufand times gieater than that of the lattei ; fuch aie the confequences ariing fiom the infinite divifibility of matter.

Therefoie, when the caith was in a ftate of fluidity, its component paits, folids and fluids, were uniformly

formly blended together, and thus compofed one general mafs or pulp, of equal confiftence and famenefs
in every part, from its furface to its center.

This idea of the original ftate and condition of the
terraqueous globe not only coincides with the Mofaic
account of the creation, but alfo with the opinions of
the moft ancient poets and hiftorians. They have
not indeed deduced the fubject from phyfical reafonings, but they have uniformly affeited, that the earth,
in its primitive ftate, was a confufed mafs of all things
blended together-----WITHOUT FORM---and VOID of
that order, which conftitutes bodies of different denominations, as air, water, ftones, minerals, &c.

" The Phenicians believed that the earth was origi-
" nally a fluid mafs or pulp, and the fame opinion is
" well known to have been fo ftrongly impreffed on the
" minds of the Egyptians, that one of their kings, Pto-
" lomy the fon of Lagus, is faid to have erected a tem-
" ple, in commemoration of it, built of all the various
" kinds of ftones; in which was placed an altar of
" divers colours, and a ftatue of the god Serapis, com-
" pofed of all the different metals melted together, al-
" luding to the confufion of elements." *

* See Hiftoire de la Philofophie, par Deflandes

C 2

Whether

Whether the Phenicians and Egyptians were the original authors of thofe tenets, or had borrowed them fiom the learning of more ancient nations, is not within my piovince to decide ; but according to the obfervations of Lord Bacon, on the learning of Homer and Hefiod ; may we not prefume that both thefe nations might have borrowed theii ideas on this fubject fiom the learning of moie ancient times.

The noble author writes thus, in his preface on the wifdom of the ancients. "Above all things "this prevails moft with me, and is of fingular mo-"ment ; many of thefe fables do not feem to have "been invented by the authors by whom they are ie-"lated and celebiated, as Homer, Hefiod, and others : "for if it were fo, that they took beginning in that "age, and from thofe authors by whom they are "delivered and biought to our hands, I imagine "there could be no gieat or high matter expected, "or fuppofed to proceed from them, in iefpect of "thefe oiiginals. But if with attention we confider "the matter, it will appear that they were delivered "and related as things foimerly believed and ieceiv-"ed, and not as newly invented and offered unto us. "Befides, feeing they are diveifly related by writeis "that lived near about one and the fame time, we "may

" may eafily perceive that they were common things,
" derived from precedent memorials, and that they
" became various by reafon of the divers ornaments
" beftowed on them by particular relations.

" And the confideration of this muft needs increafe
" in us a great opinion of them, as not being account-
" ed either the effects of the times or inventions of the
" poets, but as facred reliques or abftracted airs of
" better times, which, by tradition from more ancient
" nations, fell into the trumpets and flutes of the Gre-
" cians." Thus far his lordfhip.

But although we have reafon to believe that the
Egyptians and Phenicians might have received their
opinion of the chaotic ftate of the earth from more
ancient nations ; yet, as the chaos was not habitable,
this opinion could not have been merely the effect of
tradition, but the refult either of reafon or of revelation : But if this knowledge was derived from reafon,
thefe more ancient nations have probably been ac-
quainted with fome of the principles of the Newtonian
philofophy, as the chaotic ftate of the earth could not
be deduced from any other doctrines yet difcovered.

CHAP.

CHAP. III.

*Of the Chaos, whether it was instantaneous or pro-
gressively formed into an habitable World.*

No one can doubt but that the same BEING who
created matter, and governs it by immutable laws,
could have formed the chaos into an habitable world
in a moment of time, had he so pleased.

It is not, however, the business of Philosophy to inquire what the DEITY might have done in the formation of the earth ; but to deduce from the phenomena
of Nature, by what mode he has chosen to act in con-
tinuation and government of his works : for since the
laws of Nature are immutable, it seems to follow, that
by whatever mode the operations of Nature are daily
carried on, by the same mode the chaotic mass was
formed into an habitable world.

A little reflection will shew, that no instantaneous
productions either in the animate or inanimate worlds,
ever occur to our observation.

The plants and fruits of the earth rise to maturity
from their seeds, or first principles, in a regular uniform
progression : and we have many instances of the pro-

I   gressive

greffive formation of ftone, mineials, &c. in the bowels of the eaith ; and fome of them very obvious.

1. The fprings at Matlock-Bath in Derbyfhiie, tho'
extiemely pellucid and friendly to the human conftitution, are neverthelefs plentifully faturated with calca-
iious matter, which readily adheres to vegetables and
other fubftances immerfed in their ftreams, and thus,
by a conftant accietion, large maffes of ftone are gia-
dually formed. The banks on which the bath-houfes
ftand, and likewife the buildings themfelves, aie moftly compofed of fuch materials.

2. The lime-ftone *ftrata* in Deibyfhire, and many
other parts of England, abound with the *exuviæ*
of marine animals, oi the impreffions of them, in the
folid fubftance of the ftone ; and we have likewife
feveial inftances ielated by authors, of the bones of
terieftrial animals, and alfo of wood, having been
found inveloped in *ftrata* of ftone

Thus " a complete human fkeleton, with Biitifh
" beads, chains, iion iings, biafs bitts of biidles, &c.
" were dug up in a ftone-quaiiy, neai the Earl of
" Widiington's feat, at Blankney in Lincolnfhiie."

Human bones and aimoui, with Roman coin, *fibu-*
læ, &c. weie found in a ftone-pit, in the paik at Hun-
flanton,.

ftanton, in Norfolk, fuppofed to have been buried in the earth after a battle. Baddan's Abridg. Philof. Tranf. vol. vi. p. 444.

In the mountains of Canne, half a league from Meaftrick, the *vertebræ* of a crocodile, thirty feet long, was found in a *ftratum* of fand-ftone, well preferved. See Monthly Review, vol. l pag 619.

3. The beds of argillaceous ftone, &c. incumbent on coal, contain a great variety of figured foffils, reprefenting different fpecies of the vegetable creation.

Phenomena of this nature plainly evince that all fuch beds of ftone muft have been originally in a ftate of fluidity, to receive the bodies thus entombed : therefore corroborate the refult of chap. I.

4. The conftant accumulation of mineral fubftances in the caverns and fiffures of the lime-ftone *ftrata* is no lefs evident than the ftony concretions. The ftalactites which hang from their roofs, as icicles from the eves of houfes, are continually increafing in magnitude ; and the bottoms and fides of the caverns are daily incrufting with fpar, and other mineral fubftances. Such operations of Nature may be conveniently obferved in that celebrated cavern called Pool's Hole, near Buxton.

5. Many

5. Many of thefe fubterraneous caverns and fiffures are incrufted with alternate *laminæ* of fpar, lead ore, zinc ore, pyrites, &c. and here thefe bodies cryftalize, according to the nature of their component parts. Were we allowed to reafon upon the genctal caufe of thefe wonderful operations, we fhould be apt to conclude, from the appearances of them, that they are carried on by means of water filtrating flowly through the incumbent lime-ftone *ftrata*, and taking up in its paffage a variety of heterogeneous fubftances. The water being thus faturated with mineral particles, enters the caverns and fiffures in a quiefcent ftate, where the aqueous particles evaporate, and leave the metalic ones to unite, according to their affinities. Hence a variety of mineral bodies are daily forming.

Now fince it appears that the operations of Nature are progreffive in the formation of ftones and minerals of various denominations ; and not only in thefe inftances, but univerfally, fo far as human reafon has hitherto been able to trace them ; therefore, the prefumption is great, that the earth was brought to maturity from a chaotic mafs, by the fame univerfal laws, in a regular, uniform progreffion.

D

CHAP.

ftanton, in Norfolk, fuppofed to have been buried in the earth after a battle. Baddan's Abridg. Philof. Tranf. vol. vi. p. 444.

In the mountains of Canne, half a league from Meaftrick, the *vertebræ* of a crocodile, thirty feet long, was found in a *ftratum* of fand-ftone, well preferved. See Monthly Review, vol. l. pag 619.

3. The beds of argillaceous ftone, &c. incumbent on coal, contain a great variety of figured foffils, re-piefenting different fpecies of the vegetable cieation.

Phenomena of this nature plainly evince that all fuch beds of ftone muft have been originally in a ftate of fluidity, to receive the bodies thus entombed : there-foie coiroborate the refult of chap. I.

4. The conftant accumulation of mineral fubftan-ces in the caveins and fiffures of the lime-ftone *ftrata* is no lefs evident than the ftony concretions. The ftalactites which hang fiom theii ioofs, as icicles fiom the eves of houfes, are continually increafing in magnitude ; and the bottoms and fides of the caverns aie daily incrufting with fpai, and other mineial fub-ftances. Such opeiations of Nature may be conve-niently obfeived in that celebrated cavern called Pool's Hole, near Buxton.

5. Many

5. Many of thefe fubterraneous caverns and fiffuies are inciufted with alternate *laminæ* of fpar, lead oie, zinc oie, pyrites, &c. and here thefe bodies cryftalize, according to the nature of their component parts. Were we allowed to reafon upon the geneial caufe of thefe wonderful opeiations, we fhould be apt to conclude, from the appearances of them, that they aie carried on by means of water filtiating flowly through the incumbent lime-ftone *ftrata*, and taking up in its paffage a vaiiety of heterogeneous fubftances. The water being thus faturated with mineral particles, enters the caverns and fiffures in a quiefcent ftate, where the aqueous paiticles evapoiate, and leave the metalic ones to unite, according to their affinities. Hence a vaiiety of mineral bodies are daily foiming.

Now fince it appears that the opeiations of Natuie are progreffive in the formation of ftones and mineials of various denominations ; and not only in thefe inftances, but univeifally, fo fai as human ieafon has hitheito been able to tiace them , theiefoie, the piefumption is great, that the eaith was biought to matuiity from a chaotic mafs, by the fame univerfal laws, in a regular, unifoim progieflion.

D   C H A P.

CHAP. IV.

An Inquiry whether the component Parts of the Chaos were created homogeneous or heterogeneous.

ACcording to the preceding chapters, the terraqueous globe was originally a fluid, chaotic mafs, and progreffively formed into an habitable world : therefore let us now inquire whether its component parts were created homogeneous or heterogeneous.

If the former, according to the immutable laws of Nature, they muft have remained of one univerfal denomination, affinity, or famenefs, to the end of time.

On the contrary, if they were created heterogeneous, or endued with different qualities, affinities, or laws of attraction, they muft, in like manner, neceffarily remain of contrary affinities or qualities, to the end of time.

That the component parts of the earth are heterogeneous, or governed by different laws of attraction, is a felf-evident truth : therefore, fince thofe laws are immutable, it feems reafonable to conclude, that the component parts of the chaos were *heterogeneous*, or endued with peculiar laws of attraction ; though

equally

equally governed by *one* and the fame law of univerfal gravitation.

Now fince it appeals, that the component parts of
the chaos were endued with different laws of attraction, it becomes neceffary to inveftigate thefe laws, as
they are of fingular moment in the explanation of natural phenomena, and effentially different fiom the at-
tracftion of giavitation.   The celebiated chymift, M.
Macquer, has, I think, fet thefe matters in a veiy clear
light : viz.

" All experiments hitheito made, concur with daily
" obfervation, to prove that diffeient bodies, whether
" principles or compounds, have fuch a mutual con-
" foimity, ielation, affinity, oi attiacftion if you will
" call it fo, as difpofes fome of them to join and unite
" together, while they aie incapable of contiacfting
" any union with otheis.   This effecft, whatever be
" its caufe, will enable us to account for, and connecft
" together, all the phenomena that chymiftry pro-
" duces.   The natuie of this univeifal affecftion of
" matter is diftincftly laid down in the following pio-
" pofitions.

" Fiift, If one fubftance has any affinity oi confoi-
" mity to another, the two will unite together, and
" foim one compound.

D 2   " Secondly,

" Secondly, It may be laid down as a general rule,
" that all fimilar fubftances have an affinity with
" each other, and are confequently difpofed to unite,
" as water with water, earth with earth, &c.

" Thirdly, Subftances that unite together, lofe fome
" of their feparate properties, and the compounds re-
" fulting from their union partake of the properties of
" thofe fubftances which ferve as their principles.

" Fourthly, The fimpler any fubftances are, the
" more perceptible and confiderable are their affini-
" ties : whence it follows, that the lefs bodies are
" compounded, the more difficult it is to analyze
" them ; that is, to feparate from each other, the
" principles of which they confift.

" Fifthly, If a body confift of two fubftances, and
" to this compound be prefented a third fubftance,
" that has no affinity at all with one of the two pri-
" mary fubftances aforefaid, but has a greater affinity
" to the other than thofe two fubftances have to each
" other, there will enfue a decompofition, and a new
" union : that is, the third fubftance will feparate
" the two compounding fubftances from each other,
" coalefce with that which has an affinity with it,
" form therewith a new combination, and difengage,
" the

" the other which will then be left at liberty, and
" such as it was before it had contracted any union.

" Sixthly, It happens sometimes, that when a third
" substance is presented to a body, consisting of two
" substances, no decomposition follows ; but the two
" compounding substances, without quitting each
" other, unite with the substance presented to them,
" and form a composition of three principles , and
" this comes to pass when the third substance has
" equal, or nearly equal, affinity with each of the
" compounding substances. The same thing may
" also happen, even when the third substance hath no
" affinity but with one of the compound substances
" only. To produce such an effect, it is sufficient
" that one of the two compounding substances have
" to the third body a relation equal, or nearly equal,
" to that which it has to the other compounding sub-
" stance with which it is already combined. Thence
" it follows, that two substances, which, when apart
" from all others, are incapable of contracting any
" union, may be rendered capable of incorporat-
" ing together in some measure, and becoming parts
" of the same compound, by combining with a third
" substance, with which each of them has an equal
" affinity.

Seventhly,

" Seventhly, A body which of itfelf cannot de-
" compofe a compound confifting of two fubftances,
" becaufe, as we juft now faid, they have a greater
" affinity with each other than it has with either of
" them, becomes neverthelefs capable of feparating
" the two by uniting with one of them, when it is
" itfelf combined with any other body, having a de-
" gree of affinity with that one fufficient to compen-
" fate its own want thereof.   In that cafe, there will
" be two affinities, and thence enfues a double de-
" compofition, and a double combination." See M.
Macquer's Elements of Chymiftry, vol. i. p. 11, 12,
13, 14.

Such are the conftant invariable laws impreffed upon matter, from the beginning of the world to the
prefent time , whence many phenomena in the great
fyftem of Nature feem to arife.

CHAP.

CHAP. V.

Of the Separation of the Chaos into Air, Water, &c.

HAVING premifed the general laws or principles beftowed upon matter, let us endeavour to trace their operations in forming the chaotic mafs into an habitable world.

The firft operation which prefents itfelf to our conception is the figure of the earth : for according to propofition the fecond, the fluid mafs no fooner began to revolve upon its axis, than its component parts began to recede from their axes of motion, and thus continued till the two forces were equally balanced, and the earth had acquired its prefent oblate fpheroidical form.

The component parts being now arrived at a ftate of reft, with refpect to the general laws of motion,* began a fecond operation by means of their affinities; for, according to prop. 2, pag. 21, particles of a fimilar nature attract each other more powerfully than thofe of a contrary affinity or quality.

* See propofitions 1ft and 2d, pag 4, and 6.

Hence

Hence particles of air united with thofe of air ; thofe of watei with water ; and thofe of earth with earth ; and with their union commenced their fpecific gravities.

The unifoim fufpenfion of the component parts being thus deftioyed by the union of fimilar particles, thofe bodies which were the moft denfe began their appioach towards the center of gravity, and the others towaids the furface.

Thus commenced the feparation of the chaotic mafs into *air*, *water*, *earth*, &c.

Now as *air* is eight hundred times lighter than watei, it feems to follow, by the laws of ftatics, that it became freed from the geneial mafs in a like proportion of time, foonei than water, and formed a *muddy, impure atmofphere*.

The piocefs of feparation ftill goes on, and the earth confolidates eveiy day moie and moie towaids its centie, and its furface becomes gradually covered with watei, until one *univerfal fea* prevailed over the globe, peifectly *pure* and *fit* for *animal life*.

Thus, by the union of fimilar paiticles, the component paits of the atmofphere and the ocean feem to have been fepaiated from the geneial mafs, affembled together, and furrounded the teiraqueous globe.

I   To

To the peculiar laws of attraction may likewife be afcribed that famenefs of quality which prevails in *ftrata* of different denominations, as calcarious, argil-laceous, &c. and alfo the affemblage of all other particles into felect bodies, of metals, minerals, falts, talks, fpars, fluors, cryftals, diamonds, rubies, amethyfts, &c. and many other phenomena in the natural world.

Having thus defined the general laws or principles by which the component parts of the chaos were feparated and arranged into the different claffes of air, water, &c. it may not be improper to remark, that as the fun is the common center of gravity or the governing principle in the planetary fyftem, the prefumption is great that the governing body was at leaft co-eval with the bodies governed :

Therefore, as the chaos revolved upon its axis during the feparation of its component parts, may we not thence infer, that as the atmofphere was progreffively freed from its grofs matter, light and heat muft have gradually increafed, until the fun became vifible in the firmament, and fhone with its full luftre and brightnefs on the face of the new-formed globe.

Hence it appears, that feveral days and nights preceded the fun's appearance in the heavens. How far the refult of this reafoning may illuftrate the Mofaic

account

account, of the fun being created, or becoming vifible, on the fourth day of creation, is moſt humbly ſubmitted to the confideration and candour of the learned world.

It is further to be obſerved, that as the ſeparation of the chaos was owing to the union of ſimilar particles, it ſeems to follow, that as the central parts of the eaith were ſooner at reſt than the more ſuperficial parts thereof, that the former would begin to confolidate befoie the latter, and therefore it appears repugnant to the laws of Nature, that the central part ſhould confiſt of water only, and the more ſuperficial part of a ſhell or ciuſt, as ſome writers have imagined.

C H A P.

CHAP. VI.

On the Formation of the primitive Iſlands.

HAving tiaced the operations of Nature in ſeparating the chaotic maſs into air, eaith, and water, we have now to inquire into the formation of the primitive iſlands.

To inveſtigate this matter, let us ſuppoſe, for the preſent, that during the ſeparation of the chaos, the earth was peifeƈtly fiee fiom the attiaƈtive influence of all other bodies , that nothing inteifeied with the unifoim law of its own gravitation. It will then follow, that as the chaos was an unifoim pulp, the folids would equally fubfide fiom eveiy pait of its furface, and confequently become equally coveied with watei.

On the contiaiy, if the moon was coeval with the eaith, its attiaƈtive power would gieatly inteifeie with the uniform fubfiding of the folids : for as the feparation of the folids and fluids incieaſed, fo, in like manner, the tides would increaſe, and remove the folids about, fiom place to place, without any order or regularity.

Hence

Hence, the fea neceffarily became unequally deep, and thofe inequalities daily increafing, in procefs of time dry land would appear, and divide the fea, which had univerfally covered the earth.

The primitive iflands being thus raifed, by the flux and reflux of the tides, as fand-banks are formed in the fea, we cannot fuppofe them to have been of any great extent or elevation, compared to the mountains and continents in the prefent ftate of the earth : therefore they can only be confidered as fo many protuberances gradually afcending from the deep : whence it appears, that craggy rocks and impending fhores were not then in being ; all was fmooth, even, and uniform ; ftones, minerals, &c. only exifted in their elementary principles.

The primitive iflands being thus raifed above the furface of the fea, in procefs of time, became firm, and fit for animal or vegetable life.

Having now confidered the formation of the atmofphere, the fea and the land, I cannot pafs over in filence the great analogy between the Mofaic account of the creation and the refult of phyfical reafonings, in fo many effential points : for we find the fame feries of truths afferted in Scripture which are here deduced from the univerfal laws and operations of Nature.

From

From this obvious agreement of revelation with reafon, may we not conclude, that they both flow from
the fame fountain, and therefore cannot operate in
contradiction to each other ? Confequently, by which
ever means the fame truths are brought to light, be it
by *reafon* or *revelation*, they will perfectly coincide,
and that coincidence may be confidered as a teftimony of the truth of each.

CHAP.

C H A P. VII.

Of the Creation of marine Animals, and of their be-
ing entombed in the Bowels of the Earth.

THE atmofphere, fea and land, being now arrived
at a ftate of maturity for the reception of the animal
and vegetable kingdoms, it becomes neceffary to inquire into the order or fucceffion in which the different fpecies were created.

It has already been obferved, chap. v. that the earth
in its primitive ftate was univerfally covered with water, which became perfectly pure and fit for animal
life, before the iflands were formed, for the reception
of terreftrial animals.

To inveftigate thefe matters, let us fuppofe, for the
prefent, that marine animals were created during the
univerfality of the ocean ; this being granted, it feems
to follow, that as the marine inhabitants *increafe* and
multiply exceedingly, they would replenifh the whole
extent of the fea, from pole to pole, in a fhort fpace of
time.

The waters being thus ftocked with inhabitants before the primitive iflands were formed, many of thefe

I   animals

animals muft neceffarily become inveloped and buried in the mud, while the iflands were raifing See chap. vi. Hence it follows, that the deeper the primitive ocean, the longer the iflands were in forming, and the deeper thefe animal bodies were entombed.

Thefe matters being granted, it feems to follow, that as marine animals are endued with different degrees of activity, thofe which are the leaft active, would confequently be the leaft able to defend themfelves from fuch interments : therefore, as all fpecies of fhell-fifh are lefs active than the finny kinds, the former were confequently buried in greater numbers than the latter.

Such are the confequences arifing from the marine animals being created prior to the formation of the primitive iflands. Whence it follows,

1. That as the fea univerfally prevailed over the earth, and was univerfally inhabited, confequently many of thofe inhabitants muft have been buried in all parts of the fea, from pole to pole.

2. And if they were buried and deprived of life in fucceffive periods of time, they muft confequently be found at different depths in the earth ; in different ftates of decay, and different ftates of petrefaction.

Having

Having proceeded thus far hypothetically it becomes neceffary to inquire into the phenomena which relate to the *exuviæ* of marine animals found in the earth, and to obferve their analogy with the preceding conclufions : for on their agreement, the refult of this reafoning muft ftand or fall.

It is a truth univerfally known, that all parts of the world hitherto explored abound with the *exuviæ* of marine animals, as the bones, teeth, and fhells of fifh, embodied in the folid fubftance of ftone, chalk, clay, &c. and that, in all thefe beds the fragments of fea fhells are infinitely more numerous than the bones or teeth of fifh ; and that the latter are generally found near the furface, blended with a variety of adventitious bodies. On the contrary, fhell-fifh are found at the depth of many hundred yards, embodied in the folid fubftance of the lime-ftone *ftrata*, through their whole thicknefs , as may be obferved in all the cliffs, and in the deepeft mines in Derbyfhire. See the Appendix.

The fame phenomena likewife abound in various parts of Staffordfhire, Shropfhire, Nottinghamfhire, Leicefterfhire, &c.

1. And, according to M. Buffon, " foffil fhells are " found in the Alps, on the top of mount Cenis, in the " Appenines, in the mountains of Genoa, and in moft
                                                    " of

" of the quarries of ftone and marble in Italy ; in moft
" parts of Germany and Hungary, and indeed gene-
" rally in all the elevated places in Europe. We al-
" fo find them in the ftones whereof the moft ancient
" edifices of the Romans were conftructed.

2. " In Switzerland, Afia and Africa, travellers
" have obferved petrified fifh, in many places : for in-
" ftance, on the mountains of Caftravan, there is a bed
" of white laminated ftone, and each lamina contains
" a great number and diverfity of fifhes ; they are,
" for the moft part, very flat, and extremely compref-
" fed, in the manner of foffil fern , yet they are fo
" well preferved, that the minuteft marks of their fins
" and fcales are diftinguifhable, and every other part,
" whereby one fpecies of fifh is known from another.

3. " There are likewife many *echenites* and pe-
" trified fifh between Iver and Cairo, and on all the
" hills and heights of Barbary, moft of which exactly
" correfpond with the like fpecies taken in the Red
" Sea.

4. " The long chain of mountains, which extend
" from eaft to weft, from the lower part of Portugal
" quite to the moft eaftern parts of China, thofe
" which ftretch collaterally to the north and fouth of
" them, together with the mountains of Africa and

F   Ame-

" America, which are now known to us, all contain
" *strata* of earth and stone, full of shells.

5. " The islands of Europe, Asia, and America,
" wherein Europeans have had occasion to dig, whe-
" ther in mountains or plains, all furnish us with shells,
" and convince us that they have this particular in
" common with their adjacent continents.

6. " The *glossoptra*, or the teeth of sharks, and
" of other fishes, are found in the jaws, polished and
" worn smooth at the extremities ; consequently must
" have been made use of during the animal's life ;
" and in the shells, the very pearls are found, which
" the living animals of the same kind produce.

7. " It is well known that the *purpura* and *pho-*
" *lades* have a long pointed proboscis, which serves
" them as a kind of gimblet or drill, to pierce the
" shells of living fish, on whose flesh they feed. Now
" shells thus pierced are found in the earth, which is
" another incontestible proof that they heretofore in-
" closed living fish, and that these fish inhabited places
" where the *purpura* and *pholades* preyed on them.

8. " In Holland sea shells are found an hundred
" feet below the surface ; at Merly-la-Ville, six leagues
" from Paris, at seventy-five ; and in the Alps and Py-
                                        " renean

‘ renean mountains they are found under beds of ftone
‘ of an hundred, nay even a thoufand feet.

9. " Shells are likewife found in the mountains of
‘ Spain, France, and England ; in all the marble quar-
‘ ries in Flanders ; in the mountains of Guilders ; in
‘ all the hills round Paris ; in thofe of Burgundy and
‘ Champagne ; and, in fhort, in all places where the
‘ bafis of the foil is neither *freeftone* nor *fandftone*.

10. " By fhells I would be undeiftood to mean, not
‘ only thofe which are merely teftaceous, but the re-
‘ licks of the cruftaceous fifhes alfo ; and even all
‘ other maiine produdtions : and I can venture to
‘ affert, that in the geneiality of marbles there is fo
‘ great a quantity of maiine produdtions, that they
‘ appear to furpafs in bulk the matter wheieby they
‘ are united.

11. " Amongft the many inftances of the multipli-
‘ city of oyfters, there are few more extraordinaiy
‘ than that immenfe bed which M. de Reaumui gives
‘ an account of, which contains 130,630,000 cubic
‘ fathoms.

12. " This vaft mafs of marine bodies is in Tou-
‘ iaine in France, at upwards of thirty-fix leagues
‘ from the fea. Some of thefe fhells aie found fo in-

F 2   " tue,

" tire, that their different fpecies are very diftinguifh-
" able.

13. " Some of the fame pieces are found recent on
" the coaft of Poictou, and others are known to be na-
" tives of more diftant parts of the world.   Amongft
" them aie likewife blended fome fragments of the
" more ftony kinds of fea plants, fuch as *madripores,*
" *fungi marini, &c.*   The canton of Touraine con-
" tains full nine fquare leagues in furface, and fur-
" nifhes thefe fragments of fhells, wherever you dig.".
Thus far M. Buffon.   See his Natural Hiftory.

14. " We fhall, however, be lefs aftonifhed at this
" very confiderable quantity of fhells, when we con-
" fider the vaft increafe of fhell fifh.   It is not un-
" common to take away a bed of thefe fhell fifh, fe-
" veral fathoms in thicknefs ; and though the places
" where they are fifhed for appear to be intirely ex-
" haufted, yet, in the enfuing year, there fhall be as
" many found in all thefe places as befoie : nor do
" I remembei to have heard that any place whence
" they weie taken, had ever been intirely exhaufted.

15. " Near Reading in Beikfhire, a continued bo-
" dy of oyfter- fhells has been found ; they lie in a
" *ftratum* of greenifh fand, about two feet in thick-
" nefs, and extend ovei five or fix acres of ground ;
                                                " they

" they are covered by *ſtrata* of ſand and clay, up-
" wards of fourteen feet deep : ſeveral whole oyſteis
" are found with both their valves or ſhells lying to-
" gether, as oyſters before they are opened ; the
" ſhells are very brittle, and in digging them up, one
" of the valves will frequently drop from its fellow.
" Several are dug out entiie ; nay ſome double oy-
" ſters, with their valves united." Lowthorp's Abr.
Phil. Tranſ. vol. ii. p. 428.

16. " In a quarry at the eaſt end of Broughton in
" Lincolnſhire, innumerable fragments of the ſhells of
" ſhell fiſh, of various ſorts, are found under a *ſtra-*
" *tum* of ſtone embodied in clay, with pieces of co-
" ral, and ſometimes whole ſhell fiſh, with their natu-
" ral ſhells and colours : ſome are moſt miſerably
" cracked, biuiſed and broken ; others totally ſqueez-
" ed flat by the incumbent weight of earth." Lowthorp's Abr. Phil. Tranſ. vol. ii. p. 428.

17. " Shaiks teeth are dug up in the iſle of Shep-
" pey, retaining their natuial colour not petrified.

18. " The *gloſſopetra*, or ſharks teeth, have like-
" wiſe been taken out of a rock in Hindeiſkelf Paik,
" near Malton in Yorkſhire." Lowthorp's Abridg.
Phil. Tranſ. vol. ii. p. 430.

19. " In

19. " In the ifle of Caldey, and elfewhere about
" Tenby in Pembrokefhire, marine foffils have been
" found in folid marble, on the face of the broken
" fea cliffs, *two hundred fathoms* below the *upper fur-*
" *face of the rocks.* Nor were they only obferved
" upon the face of thefe rocks, but even more or lefs
" throughout the whole mafs or extent of them.

" This is manifeft from divers rocks hewn down by
" workmen for making of lime, and other pieces ca-
" fually fallen from the cliffs.

20. " Thoufands of foffil teeth, exactly anfwering
" to thofe of divers forts of fea fifh, have been
" found in quarries and gravel pits, about Oxford."
Ray, 3 Dif. p. 178. 182.

21. " At Thame in Oxfordfhire, the *belemnites,* or
" thunderbolt ftones, are found in a *ftratum* of blue
" clay, which ftill retain their *native fhelly fubftance.*

22. " The *belemnites* found in gravel pits, have
" fuffered much, by their being rubbed againft each
" other in the fluctuation of waters.

23. " The *nautili* and *belemnites* are frequently
" found at Garfing near Oxford." Philof. Tranfact.
vol. liv. p. 5.

24. " At Weftbere, an obfcure village, about three
" miles eaft of Canterbury, many oyfters and other
" fhells

' fhells were dug up, at a confiderable depth, toge-
' ther with an *iron anchor :* and another anchor was
' dug at Broom Down, on the fame fide the level.

25. " Hardel Cliff, in Hampfhire, contains a great
' variety of turbinated and bivalve fhells, which ftill
' retain the native matter and colour of marine fhells ;
' many of thefe are natives of very diftant regions,
' and others of them are not known to exift in a liv-
' ing ftate.

26. " In fome parts of Suffolk, I am told, foffil
' fhells are fo numerous, that they are dug up for ma-
' nure, and produce excellent crops. Thefe fhells
' retain much of their native marine matter ; they are
' much decayed and blunted, as fhells by rolling on
' the fea coaft.

27. " Sheppey Ifle, and other parts of Kent, abound
' with foffil fhells, which ftill retain their native co-
' lour and confiftence ; likewife the teeth and *verte-*
' *bræ* of fifh, and, in particular, thofe of the fhark ;
' alfo the remains of cruftaceous fifhes, as crabs, lob-
' fters, &c.

28. " In a hill called Catfgrove, in Berkfhire, a
' great number of oyfters are dug up entire, but crum-
' ble into duft, when expofed to the air. In the fame
" place

I

" place are alfo found periwinkle fhells, whofe fpirals
" are reverfed to thofe in the adjacent fea.

29. " Rungwell Hill, in Surry, is faid to contain
" oyfter fhells not petrified, nor much decayed, and fo
" like to oyfters newly taken from the fea, that they
" have been opened for fuch, in expectation of find-
" ing living fifh therein." Ray 3 Dif. p. 129.

30. Near Stableford, the feat of the Earl of Harbo-
rough, feveral beds of fea fhells were lately difcovered,
inclofed in calcarious earth ; thefe fhells ftill retain
their native marine matter, though much decayed.
The limeftone *ftrata* in that neighbourhood abound
with different fpecies of foffil fhells, in a petrified
ftate.

31. Many parts of Northamptonfhire contain foffil
fhells, in great abundance, in part and wholly petrified,
and, in particular, a fpecies of oyfter, faid to be a native of the Mediterranean Sea. I have in my poffeffion a fragment of a *Cornu-Ammonis*, dug up near
Northampton, which retains its native fhell.

In Mr. Lever's excellent Mufeum, are two curious
fpecimens of the *Cornu-Ammonis*, with their native
fhelly matter remaining : fuch inftances are rare, and
of great value, by pointing out the origin of them.

32. " In fome parts of Virginia, for feveral miles
" together, the foil is fo intermixed with oyfter fhells,
" that there feems to be as great a quantity of fhells
" as of earth : how deep they lie thus intermixed, I
" think, is not yet known ; for in the broken banks
" they are continued many yards perpendicular. In
" feveral places the fhells are much clofer, and being
" petrified, feem to form a *ftratum* of ftone. I have
" feen, in feveral places, veins of thefe rocky fhells,
" three or four yards thick, at the foot of an hill,
" whofe perpendicular height might be twenty or
" thirty yards. Of thefe rocks of oyfter fhells that
" are not fo much petrified, they burn and make all
" their lime.

" Often in the loofer banks of fhells and earth, are
" found perfect teeth petrified, fome of them not lefs
" than two or three inches long, and above one inch
" broad ; the part that one might fuppofe to grow
" out of the jaw was polifhed, and black almoft as
" jet, the other brown, and not fo fmooth.

" The back-bone of a whale, and feveral ribs, were
" dug up out of the fide of a hill feveral yards deep,
" about four miles diftant from James-Town and the
" river. Another back-bone of a whale, and feveral
" teeth, were found in hills beyond the falls of James-

G   " River,

" River, at leaſt one hundred and fifty miles up the
" country." Lowthorp's Abrid. Phil. Tranſ. vol. iii.
p 581.

33. " Foſſil bones and ſhells of ſeveral ſorts, have
" been found in Maryland ; ſome of them have re-
" ceived little alteration in the earth, others more, and
" ſome were ſo changed as to be ſtony ; but all of
" them retained their ancient ſhape. Some of them
" were compared to the tongue and palate of a fiſh
" obſerved at Jamaica, and found perfectly analo-
" gous to each other." Lowthorp's Abridg. Philoſ.
Tranſ. vol ii. p. 431.

34. " Naphat, a remarkable mountain in Ireland,
" ſaid to be elevated ſeveral hundred fathoms above
" the level of the ſea ; yet, within ten yards of the
" top of this mountain, there are ſeveral vaſt beds of
" marine ſhells of various kinds ; as whelks, muſcles,
" cockles, &c. and parallel to theſe are thoſe vaſt
" mountains in Virginia, and other parts of America."

35. The moſt remarkable phenomenon I know, reſpecting foſſil ſhells, is at Claxby in Lincolnſhire. The
facts are as follows : It appears by a late experiment,
made by C. Pelham Eſq. of Brockleſby, for the diſco-
very of coal, that the fragments of real ſea ſhells, not
decayed, nor apparently changed from their native te-

ſtaceous

ftaceous matter, are difperfed through a *ftratum* of black indurated clay, to the depth of feventy yards : how much deeper this clay and fhells are thus continued, is not yet afcertained ; it alfo contains many nodules of iron-ftone, which are generally accompanied with a vitriolic acid, and has an incumbent *ftratum* of limeftone, which may probably be twenty or thirty yards thick. The above experiment was made where the clay *baffits* * from under the limeftone.

36. The limeftone *ftrata* in Derbyfhire contain a great variety of foffil bodies, reprefenting the *exuviæ* of marine animals, as *cockles, corals, entrochi,* &c. of various kinds, but all of them changed to a ftony fubftance. From various circumftances it appears, that thefe foffil bodies have originally, and in many inftances now lie upwards of two hundred fathoms deep. See the Appendix.

Thefe apparently marine productions are fo numerous in all parts of the world hitherto explored ; and fo univerfally obferved, that it feems needlefs to enumerate any more inftances of them : let us, therefore, confider, in a more particular manner, the phenomena

* A term ufed by miners, when an under *ftratum* appears at the furface. See the Appendix, plate I.

appertaining

appertaining to thefe foffil bodies, and proceed to draw fome general inferences concerning the origin of them.

1. The bodies thus refembling, both in fubftance and fhape, the fhells of divers forts of fhell fifh, and likewife the bones and teeth of marine animals, are found on the higheft mountains, and in parts remote from the fea ; likewife in vallies and deep receffes of the earth.

2. They are found retaining the native teftaceous matter, colour, and figure of marine fhells, infomuch as not to be diftinguifhed from the fhells of living fifh.

3. They are alfo found in various ftates of decay, and varioufly impregnated with ftony or metallic matter ; and even changed to the fubftance of the ftone in which they are inveloped.

4. They are found in the folid fubftance of lime-ftone, chalk, clay, &c. difperfed through the whole mafs of the *ftrata*, more or lefs, from their upper to their lower furfaces.

5. The bivalve fpecies are found with both their valves intire and clofe, as the fhells of living fifh ; and when they are thus found, they generally compofe di-ftinct beds of oyfters, cockles, mufcles, &c. as the fame fpecies do in the ocean.

3   6. When

6. Wherever beds confift of the fragments of fhells, I have ever found them compofed of various kinds, confufedly blended together, in like manner as the fragments of fhells are in the fea.

7. The bones and teeth refembling thofe of fifh, are alfo found, retaining the figure, colour, and polifh of recent teeth, and even apparently worn by ufe ; but though great numbers of them are found, yet the number of foffil fhells by far exceeds them.

Such are the phenomena accompanying thefe foffil bodies : therefore the following inferences may be fairly deduced.

Firft, Their analogy in fhape and fubftance to the fhells and bones of living fifh, together with a gradual change in the conftitution of their component parts, from a teftaceous fubftance to that of ftone, &c. evidently fhews, that all foffil fhells muft have been originally the productions of the fea

Secondly, their being found, in all parts of the world, on the higheft mountains, and in parts remote from the fea, plainly fhews, that the fea originally prevailed over the earth, from pole to pole, according to chap. v. and likewife, that thefe marine animals were created prior to the primitive iflands, and confequently prior to terreftrial animals, agreeable to the Scripture account.

Thirdly,

Thirdly, They are buried at various depths in the earth, and are found in various ftates of decay and degrees of petrefaction ; therefore, it feems to follow, that they were entombed, and deprived of life, in fucceffive periods of time, according to the former part of this chapter, page 30, 31.

Fourthly, Thofe which form diftinct beds of oyfters, cockles, mufcles, &c were confequently *generated*, *lived*, and *died* in the very beds wherein they were found ; and could not have been removed from diftant regions of the earth by a flood or floods of water, with fo much order as to preferve their refpective claffes diftinct or feparate from each other.

Fifthly, Their being entombed in the folid fubftance of limeftone, chalk, &c. plainly teftifies, that all fuch *ftrata* muft have been originally in a ftate of fluidity, to receive them ; according to chap. i.

The general agreement of thefe phenomena with the refult of the preceding chapters, deduced from the laws of Nature, feems to be the moft folid foundation on which general theories can be eftablifhed, or whence all real knowledge in phyfical inquiries can be truly derived.

Here it may not be improper to remark, as a further teftimony, that marine animals were created prior to

the

the primitive iflands, viz. that no terreftrial animals or vegetables are found inveloped in the limeftone *ftrata* of Derbyfhire, which contain the marine productions :* nor any remains of marine animals are ever found in the argillaceous *ftrata*, which contain the vegetable impreffions. And it is further to be obferved, that the argillaceous *ftrata*, are incumbent on the limeftone or calcareous beds : but more of this in the Appendix.

* The impreffion of a crocodile difcovered by Mr. Henry Watfon of Bakewell, near the upper furface of *ftratum* No. 3, plate I. may poffibly be confidered as an objection to that general rule.

CHAP.

C H A P. VIII.

General Observations on the superficial and interior
Parts of the Earth.

NOtwithstanding the conclusions we have drawn in
the preceding chapter, to prove the origin of fossil
shells, have so much the appearance of truth, neverthe-
less, some objections may possibly arise in the minds of
those readers who have been accustomed to consider
mountains and *continents* as *primary* productions of
Nature.   Such inquirers may probably reason thus
with themselves :

" If the fossil shells which are found in the tops of
" the highest mountains were generated, and have li-
" ved and died, in the very beds wherein they are
" found, those beds must have been originally the bot-
" tom of the ocean ; and if so, pray, whence pro-
" ceeds these vast alterations on the superficial parts
" of the earth ? Why hath the sea descended so far
" beneath those mighty eminences, the *Alps*, the *An-*
" *des*, the *Pyreneans*, &c. and why hath it retired
                                                      " from

" from thofe extenfive tracts of land, the *conti-*
" *nents ?* Were not thefe things originally thus crea-
" ted ? If not, pray whence proceeds thefe great in-
" equalities? Hiftory is filent concerning fuch events ;
" and tradition is too faint to reft much proof upon it ;
" therefore, fince we have no written evidence to
" help us in the fcrutiny, and tradition itfelf fails
" us through age, we cannot wholly affent to the
" preceding conclufions, until thefe apparent ob-
" jections are removed."

To fuch candid inquirers I beg leave to anfwer,
that whoever attentively views and confiders the prefent
fent ftate and condition of the terraqueous globe, its
craggy rocks and mountains, its fteep, angular and
impending fhores, fubterrancous caverns, &c. will be
almoft perfuaded without any farther inquiry, that
thefe romantic appearances are not the effects of a regular
gular uniform law, but of fome tremendous convulfions,
fions, which have thus burft its *ftrata,* and thrown
their fragments into all this confufion and diforder :
nay, the very reprefentation of fea and land, upon a
geographical chart, feems alone fufficient to eftablifh
the truth of fuch a conjecture.

Let us not, however, take thofe things for granted
which we are able to inveftigate from a feries of undeni-

H   niable

niable *data :* it is one thing to affert a truth, and anothei to prove it ; the former leaves the mind in a
ftate of fufpence, the latter in poffeffion of *truth.*

But before we attempt to inveftigate the caufe of
thefe wonderful appeaiances, let us endeavour to recollect the general ftate and condition of them.

We are told that " Norway abounds with ftupen-
" dous rocks and mountains, as it were, cloven afun-
" der, or cut with faws, both acrofs and lengthways.
" Some of them aie iemaikable for their appearances ;
" on the left hand, failing up Joering Creek, theie ap-
" pears fuch a group of the crefts of mountains, as re-
" femble the profpect of an old city, with toweis and
" Gothic edifices : fome of them are continually co-
" vered with fnow, whilft the chafms in others make
" way for the light to penetrate.

" The fea fhore too, is almoft every where fteep,
" angulai, and impending, infomuch that the water,
" clofe to the rocks, is geneially three or foui hun-
" died fathoms deep ; and in Floge Cicek no bottom
" can be found with a line of one thoufand fathoms.

" Noidall creek is alfo faid to be nine hundied fa-
" thoms deep ; and other creeks, which run thiity
" miles up the countiy, are alfo faid to be three or
" four hundied fathoms deep ; and the bottom of
" the

" the fea and other waters in that country confift of
" rocks, mountains, and vallies, like the land." Thus
far Bifhop Pontoppidon's Hift. of Norway.

We are alfo told, that many other parts of the
world are in a fimilar ftate to thofe of Norway.

The mountains in Derbyfhire, and the moorlands of
of Staffordfhire appear to be fo many heaps of ruins,
and more efpecially the latter; for, in the neighbourhood of Ecton, Wetton, Dovedale, Ilam, and Switham-
ly, the *ftrata* lie in the utmoft confufion and difordei.
They aie broken, diflocated, and thrown into every
poffible direction, and their interior paits aie no lefs
rude and romantic, for they univeifally abound with
fubteiraneous caverns; and, in fhort, with every poffible mark of violence. The caveins near Buxton and
Caftleton, and the fubterraneous riveis, the Manifold
and the Hamps, are familiai inftances of the prefent
ftate and condition of thofe paits of the globe. The
former iiver, after a paffage of foui oi five miles fiom
the noith, and the latter about the fame diftance fiom
the weft both emerge at the foot of the fame cliff, in
the gaden of John Poit, efq. of Ilam, about the diftance of twenty yards from each other.

We may add, to the above obfeivations, that extraordinaiy phenomenon of laige blocks of ftone being

feattered

scattered over the surface of mountainous countries, and blended with their soils to very considerable depths, as if they had been originally ejected from their native beds by subterraneous blasts, as stones from Vesuvius and Ætna.

The fragments are thus circumstanced : those which lie near their native beds are too numerous and massy for the hand of man to have placed them there, and are in as much disorder as stones casually thrown together. The banks on the east side of the river Derwent, from Crich Cliff, for twenty miles up the river, are thus covered ; and the same may be said of many other mountains in Derbyshire and Staffordshire.

These stones lying so near their original *stratum*, we may easily satisfy ourselves that they are detached parts thereof ; and, by analogy, the more distant fragments may be ascertained with equal certainty, tho' at the distance of ten or twenty miles.

In the neighbourhoods of Utoxeter, in Staffordshire, blocks of limestone are frequently dug up, of four or five hundred weight each , and yet I cannot learn that there are any quarries of the same kind nearer than four or five miles.

The fragments of stone perfectly analogous to the former, were dug up at Etwall in Derbyshire. A well
being

being funk, to the depth of eleven yards, many of thefe ftones were found, intermixed with other adventitious bodies, from the furface of the earth to that depth, fome of them were fix or eight pounds weight, and fome fmaller. Now although Etwall cannot be lefs than fifteen or twenty miles from any known quarry of the fame kind, we cannot help concluding that they were originally ejected to that diftance; fince fuch effects are frequently produced by fubterraneous explofions : and what makes this conjecture more probable, the fame phenomena have been obferved in many other wells in that village.

I have alfo feen many blocks of Cornifh Moor-ftone, or granite, in feveral parts of Staffordfhire and Shropfhire, and particularly in the neigbourhood of Newport.

The preceding inftances may ferve to fhew the general ftate and condition of the terraqueous globe : therefore we have now to inquire what alterations have been produced on the fuperficial parts of the earth fince the commencement of hiftory, in order to obferve the analogy between thofe effects, and the appearances we have been enumerating, which is referved for the fubject of the enfuing chapter.

CHAP.

CHAP. IX.

*On the Alterations produced on the superficial Parts of
the Earth since the Commencement of History, by
subterraneous Convulsions.*

WE learn from Pliny and other natural historians,
that the superficial parts of the earth have suffered
great alterations, at different periods of time, viz.

1. That many mountains have been raised, and
others depressed, or totally swallowed, with cities, and
large districts of land ; and that navigable lakes have
appeared in the places of them.

2. That many mountains have likewise been shivered to pieces, and their fragments thrown into their
adjacent vallies, and even to the distance of ten or fifteen miles.

3. That great clefts or fissures have been frequently
produced, from whence rivers of water and melted
matter have flowed, and deluged the adjacent countries , and likewise that great agitations of the sea,
and also rivers, and lakes in the inland countries, have
frequently accompanied these tremendous convulsions
of Nature.

Let

Let us, therefore, first, recite a few recent instances, to strengthen the credibility of those which happened in the more early ages of the world.

1. We are told, that in the dreadful earthquake, which destroyed Lisbon, on the first of November 1755, " the mountains of Arrabida, Estretta, Julio, Marvan, " and Cintra, being some of the largest in Portugal, " were impetuously shaken as it were to their very " foundations, and some of them opened at their " summits, split, and rent in a wonderful manner, and " huge masses of them were thrown down into the ad- " jacent vallies."*

" A fine new stone quay, where the merchants land " their goods, where at that time about three thousand " people were assembled for safety, was turned bottom " upwards, and every one perished : nor did so much " as a single body appear afterwards."† I have since been credibly informed, that the water where the quay stood is now one hundred fathoms deep.

2 " A sea port, called St. Ubal's, was intirely " swallowed up, people and all."‡

3. " In Morocco, the earth opened, and swallowed " up a village with all its inhabitants, to the number of

---

* See Hist & Philos of Earthquakes, p 317.
† Philos. Transf vol. xlix p. 412. ‡ Ibid, p 413.

" eight

" eight or ten thoufand perfons, together with their
" cattle of all forts, as camels, horfes, horned cattle,
" &c. and foon after the caith clofed again, in the
" fame manner as it was before."*

4. " The famous city Taffo was wholly fwal-
" lowed , no remains being left."†

5. " One of the Sarjon Hills was rent in two; one
" fide of which fell upon a large town, where there
" was the famous fanctuary of their prophet, known
" by the name of Mula Teiis ; and the other fide of
" the faid hill fell down upon another large town, and
" both towns and inhabitants were all buried under
" the faid hill. ' ‡

We have likewife many other authentic accounts of
this fatal and extenfive caithquake, in the periodical
papeis.

6. " The caithquake was moie dieadiul in Barba-
" iy than at Portugal, at Mequinez that pait of the
" city wheie the Jews iefided was intiiely fwallowed up,
" and all the people of that fect, being about four thou-
" fand in numbei, periflhed except feven or eight ||"

7. In anothei paper it is faid, " The gieat city of
" Mequinez is no moie, it was buiied in the bowels of

* Philof Trani vol. vlix p 430. | Ibid, p 432.
| Ibid, p. 431 || Gent. Mag. Jan 1756, p. 7
                2   " the

" the earth, on the nineteenth of November, by a vi-
" olent fhock of an earthquake, which likewife fwal-
" lowed up, at feveral leagues diftance, two camps
" of the moving Arabs, upward of four hundred tents,
" containing twenty-five or thirty perfons each, with
" a large tract of country."*

10. " In the year 1692, a great part of Port-Royal
" in Jamaica was funk by an earthquake, and remains
" covered by water feveral fathoms deep ; fome chim-
" nies and mafts of fhips appear above water. On the
" north fide, above 1000 acres of land funk. Some
" mountains along the river, betwixt Spanifh-Town
" and Sixteen-mile Walk were joined together ; and
" others fo thrown on heaps, that people were forced
" to go by Guanaboa to Sixteen-mile Walk.

" At Yellows, a great mountain fplit, and fell into
" the level land, and covered feveral fettlements.
" Another plantation was removed half a mile from
" the place where it formerly flood.

" In Clarendon precinct the earth gaped prodigi-
" oufly ; and all over the ifland there were abundance
" of openings, nay, many thoufands ; but in the
" mountains are faid to have been the moft violent
" fhakes : indeed they are ftrangely torn and rent,

* Gent. Mag. December 1755, p 564.

I   " infomuch

" infomuch that they feem to be of different fhapes
" now, from what they were, efpecially the Blue and
" other higheft mountains, which feem to have been
" the greateft fufferers.   And a large high mountain
" near Portmorant, near a day's journey over, is faid
" to be quite fwallowed up ; and in the place where
" it ftood there is now a great lake, of four or five
" leagues over.

" The Blue and its neighbouring mountains ufed
" to afford a fine green profpect ; now one half part
" of them at leaft feem to be wholly deprived of their
" natural verdure.   There one may fee where the
" tops of great mountains have fallen, fweeping down
" all the trees, and every thing in their way, and
" making a path quite from top to bottom." *

9. " In the year 1699, feven hills were funk by an
" earthquake, in the ifland of Java, near the head of
" the great Batavian river, five on this fide and two
" on the other.   And nine more were likewife funk
" on this fide the Tangarang river.   Between the
" Batavian and Tangarang rivers, the land was rent
" and divided afunder, with great clefts, more than a
" foot wide."†

10. " The Pico, in the Moluccos, accounted of
" equal height with that of Teneriffe, was funk by an
                                        " earth-

* Lowthorp's Abridg Phil. Tranf. vol. ii. p. 417.
† Ibid. p 419.

" earthquake, and quite fwallowed up into the earth,
" and left a lake in its place." Dr. Hooke's Poft.
p. 307.

11. " In the year 1646, many of thofe vaft moun-
" tains of the Andes were quite fwallowed up and
" loft." Dr. Hooke's Poft p. 307.

12. " In the year 1538, the famous town called St.
" Euphemia, fituate at the fide of the bay, under the
" jurifdiction of the Knights of Malta, was totally
" fwallowed up, with all its inhabitants, and nothing
" appeared but a ftinking lake in the place of it *

13. " The 11th of January, 1693, a mighty earth-
" quake happened in Sicily, and chiefly about Catanea:
" the violent dancing of the earth threatened the whole
" ifland with intire defolation. The earth opened in
" feveral places, in very long clefts, fome an hand ɔ
" breadth, others half a palm, others like great gulphs.
" In the plain of Catanea, water was thrown from
" thofe long clefts, altogether as falt as the fea.

" Great rocks were thrown down every where, and
" in the country of Lotino, a great number of people
" perifhed in the houfes beaten down by the rocks rol-
" ling down the hills. A great number of noble ftruc-
" tures lie, like a horrid defert, in vaft heaps of ruins,

* Dr. Hooke's Poft. p. 306.

I 2   " and

" and not lefs than 59,969 perfons were deftroyed by
" the fall of them, in the different parts of Sicily."*

Having enumerated a few recent inftances of the alterations produced on the fuperficial parts of the earth,
by fubterraneous convulfions, we may venture to recite
thofe which happened in the more early ages of the
world.

Pliny has not only recorded many extraordinary phenomena which happened in his own time, but has
likewife borrowed many others from the learning of
more ancient nations.

14. " A city of the Lacedemonians was deftroyed
" by an Earthquake, and its ruins wholly buried by
" the mountain Taygetus falling down upon them."
Chap. lxix. p. 37.

15. " Many ftrange effects enfue from earthquakes:
" in one place the walls of cities are laid along; in
" another they are fwallowed up in deep and wide
" chafms: here are caft up mighty heaps of earth;
" there, are let out rivers of water, and fometimes of
" fire, in another place, the courfe of rivers are
" changed. The chafms fometimes remain wide
" open, and fhew what hath been fwallowed up, at
" other times they clofe up again, and conceal all that
" is contained in them, and no vifible marks thereof

* Lowthorp's Abridg Phil. Tranf. vol. ii. p. 408, 409.

" remain,

" remain, notwithſtanding they have many times de-
" voured cities, and whole tracts of land." Pliny's
Nat. Hiſt. chap. lxx. p. 38.

16. " I found," ſays Pliny, " in the books of the
" Tuſcan learning, an earthquake recorded, which
" happened within the territory of Modena, when L.
" Martius and S. Julius were conſuls, which repeatedly
" daſhed two hills againſt each other. With this con-
" flict all the villages, and many cattle were deſtroy-
" ed ; and this happened the year before the war of
" our aſſociates : which I doubt whether it were not
" more pernicious to the whole land of Italy than the
" civil wars. This event happened in the day-time,
" and was obſerved by many Roman gentlemen.

17. " No leſs a wonder happened in our age, in
" the very laſt year of Nero the emperor ; when mea-
" dows and olive rows (notwithſtanding the great
" public port-way laid between them) paſſed into
" each others place, in the Marrucine territory." See
his Nat. Hiſt. chap. lxxiii. p. 39.

18. " The greateſt earthquake in man's memory
" was that which happened during the reign of Tibe-
" rius Cæſar, when twelve cities of Aſia were laid le-
" vel in one night." Ibid. chap. lxxiv. p. 39.

Having

19. Having recited a few inftances of *mountains,
cities*, and *large diftricts* of *land*, having been fwallowed up from time to time, in various parts of the
world ; and others which have been clove afunder,
fhivered to pieces, and their fragments thrown into
the adjacent vallies ; let us now enquire what other
effects have been produced by thefe dreadful convulfions of nature.

20. " Thofe famous iflands Delos and Rhodes are
" recorded to have grown out of the fea ; and after-
" wards thofe that were lefs, namely, Anaphe be-
" yond Melos, and Nea between Lemnus and Hel-
" lefpont. Alone, alfo, between Lebedus and Pe-
" os. Thera likewife and Therafia, among the Cy-
" clades, which firft appeared in the fourth year of the
" 135th Olympiad. Moreover among the fame
" ifles, 130 years after, Hiera : and two furlongs from
" it, after 110 years, Thia, even in our time, upon
" the eighth day before the ides of July, when M. Ju-
" nius Syllanus, and L. Balbus were confuls." Pliny's
Nat. Hift. p. 40, chap. lxxvii.

21. This truly eminent author has alfo recorded
many other confiderable alterations which have happened on the fuperficial parts of the earth, at different
periods of time ; but, for brevity fake, they are here
                            I   omitted,

omitted, being of such remote antiquity. To proceed.

22. " In the year 726 the island Hiera was enlar-
" ged to twice its former dimensions by the addition
" of another island, which united so well to it, that
" there remains no other mark of its joining than a
" cleft or fissure, which reaches from one end of the
" island to the other, and in several places is not six
" inches wide,

23. " And in the month of December, 1427, this
" island called Hiera, or the Burnt Island, was again
" increased by great rocks raised up by subterraneous
" fires. The same thing happened again in the year
" 1457: but with this difference, that the subterraneous
" fire, after having raised to the height of five or six
" feet above the water, a vast quantity of rocks,
" which formed a space about a mile in circumfe-
" rence, opened a passage for the sea water to enter,
" by which it was extinguished.

24. " In the year 1573 another island was formed,
" called the Lesser Burnt Island." Motte's Abridg.
Phil. Transf. vol. ii. p. 200. part IV.

25. " From the 24th of September to the 9th of
" October, 1650, the island of Santirinum, formerly
" called by Pliny Thera, was dreadfully shaken with
" earthquakes,

" earthquakes, fo that the inhabitants expected no-
" thing but utter ruin, and were yet more amazed to
" fee a horrid eruption of fire out of the bottom of
" the fea, about four miles to the eaftward of the·
" ifland , previous to the appearance of fire, the wa-
" ter was confiderably elevated in that place, and the
" wave fpreading itfelf round every way ; overturn-
" ed every thing it met, deftroying fhips and galleys,
" in the harbour of Candia, which was eighty miles
" diftant.

    " The eruption filled the air with afhes and horri-
" ble fulphureous vapours, and dreadful lightnings and
" thunders fucceeded.   All things in the ifland were
" covered with a yellow fulphureous cruft.   Multi-
" tudes of pumice and other ftones were thrown up,
" and carried as far as Conftantinople, and to places
" at a great diftance.   The force of this eruption was
" greateft the two firft months, when all the neigh-
" bouring fea feemed to boil ; and the volcano con-
" tinually vomited up fire-balls : upon the turning of
" the wind, great mifchief was done in the ifland of
" Santerinum ; many beafts and birds were killed :
" and on the 29th of October, and 7th of Novem-
" ber, fifty men were killed by it.   The other four
" months it lafted, tho' much abated of its former
                                          ficrcenefs,

" fiercenefs, yet it ftill caft up ftones, and feemed to
" endeavour the making of a new ifland which,
" though it do not yet perfectly appear above water,
" yet 'tis covered but eight feet by the water. It is
" alfo faid, the fea, in that place, was before fathom-
" lefs." See Dr. Hooke's Poft. Work, p. 302.

26. " In the year 1707, another ifland was difco-
" vered, where it is faid, the fea was eighty or an
" hundred fathoms deep. This ifland continually in-
" creafed in height and breadth, for the fpace of three
" years , in which time it became fix miles in circum-
" ference, and of confiderable height.' See Philof.
Tranf. vol. ii. p. 200, part iv. Motte's Abr.

27. " The ifland Santorini itfelf is faid to be com-
" pofed of burnt rocks and pumice-ftones." Ibid,
p. 200.

28. " In the year 1628, one of the iflands of the
" Azores, near the ifland of St.Michael, rofe up from
" the bottom of the fea, which, in that place, was
" 160 fathoms deep ; and this ifland, which was raif-
" ed in fifteen days, is three leagues long, a league
" and a half in breadth, and rifes 360 feet above the
" water." See Sir Wm. Hamilton's Obfervations on
Vefuvius and Ætna, p. 159.

K   29. " On

29. " On the 20th November 1720, a fubterra-
" neous fire burft out of the fea near Tercera, one
" of the Azores, which threw up fuch a vaft quantity
" of ftones, &c. in the fpace of thirty days, as formed
" an ifland about two leagues diameter, and nearly
" round.

     " Prodigious quantities of pumice-ftone and half-
" broiled fifh weie found floating on the fea, for ma-
" ny leagues round the ifland."   See Philof. Tranf.
vol. vi. part ii. p. 203.   Eames's Abr.

30. " Another example of the fame kind happened
" at Manilla one of the Philippine iflands, in the year
" 1750.   This eruption was attended with violent
" earthquakes, to which that ifland, as well as the ieft
" of the Philippines, is very much fubject."   See Rev.
Mr. Michell's Conjecture on Earthquakes, p. 16.

31. We may add to the above, the vaft quantities of
pumice-ftones, which have been fometimes found floating upon the fea, at fo great a diftance from the fhore,
as well as fiom any known volcano, that theie can be
little doubt of their being thrown up by fires fubfifting
under the bottom of the ocean.

32. " Mi. Garwin relates, that in the year 1726, a
" Dutch captain failing above eighty leagues from the
" cape of Good Hope, found the fea covered with
          I   " pumice-

" pumice-ftones, through the fpace of fix hundred
" leagues." Bertrand's Dict. of Foffils, vol. ii. p. 126.

33. " In the year 1538, a fubterraneous fire burft
" open the earth near Puzzoli, and threw up fuch a
" vaft quantity of afhes and pumice-ftones, mixed
" with water, as covered the whole country, and thus
" formed a new mountain, not lefs than three miles in
" circumference, and almoft as high as Mount Baibaro,
" near a quarter of a mile perpendicular height.

34. " Some of the afhes of this volcano reached the
" vale of Diana, and fome parts of Calabria, which are
" more than 150 miles from Puzzoli." See Sir Wm.
Hamilton's Obfervat. on Ætna and Vefuvius, p. 128.

35. The few inftances we have related of iflands
being raifed in the ocean by fubteiraneous fires, ftreng-
then our conjectures concerning the origin of thofe
iflands and mountains, which have a volcanic appeai-
ance, and are fuppofed to have been produced from
the fame caufe, anterior to hiftoiy, viz. Iceland, Fyal,
&c. in the Northein Sea ; St. Helena and Afcenfion
iflands, between Africa and Brafil ; Eafter or Davis's
ifland, Otaheite, &c. in the Southern Ocean ; feveral
of the Moluccas, in the Indian Sea ; Madeira, feveral
of the Azores and the Antilles, &c. in the Atlantic

K 2   Ocean ;

Ocean; the Lipari iflands, Ifchai, &c. in the Mediterranean Sea.

The above may ferve to put the reader in mind of recollecting many other iflands which have the fame appearances; and likewife to fhew that fubterraneous fires actually exift under the bottom of the ocean, in various parts of the world; and that others may have been extinguifhed time immemorial: let us therefore return to a more particular inquiry concerning the phenomena produced by fubterraneous fires at land.

36. " In the year 1631, a ftone was thrown twelve " miles from the crater of Vefuvius, and fell upon the " Marquis of Lauro's houfe at Nola, which it fet on " fire.

37. " In the year 1767, a folid ftone, meafuring " *twelve feet* in *height*, and *forty-five* in *circumfe-* " *rence*, was thrown a quarter of a mile from the cra- " ter of Vefuvius. The eruption of 1767, though by " much the moft violent in this century, was, com- " paratively to thofe of the years 79 and 1631, very " mild." Sir Wm. Hamilton's Obfervations, p. 49.

38. " The eruption of Vefuvius, in the year 79, " overwhelmed the two famous cities Herculaneum " and Pompeii, by a fhower of ftones, cinders, afhes, " fand, &c. and totally covered them many feet deep,

3   " as

" as the people were fitting in the theatre. Her-
" culaneum is faid to have been fituate about four
" miles from the crater, and Pompeii at the diftance of
" fix miles ; yet the latter appears to have been co-
" vered by that dreadful eruption ten or fifteen feet
" deep ; and the former, by that and fubfequent
" eruptions, lies buried fixty or feventy feet deep.

" By the violence of this eruption, afhes were car-
" ried over the Mediterranean Sea, into Afiica, Egypt
" and Syria ; and at Rome they choaked the air on a
" fudden, fo as to hide the face of the fun, to the
" great terror of the inhabitants, who knew not the
" caufe thereof, having not received the news fiom
" Campania." See Burnet's Sacred Hift. vol. ii. 85, 86.

39. " In the year 1632, rocks were thiown to the
" diftance of three miles from Vefuvius."   Philof.
Tranf. vol. iii. p. 68, Baddam's Abiidg.

40. " In the year 1533, large pieces of iock were
" thrown to the diftance of thiee leagues, by the vol-
" cano Cotopaxi in Peru, and coveied the plain of La-
" tacunga ; and near Hambato the caith opened in
" feveral places, of which there ftill remains an afto-
" nifhing monument, on the fouth fide of the town,
" being a chafm oi cleft, four or five feet wide, and
" about a league in length."   See Ulloa's Voyage to
Peru, pait I. book vi.

41. " In

41. " In 1669, ftones of fixty palms in length were
" thrown fiom the crater of Ætna, to the diftance of
" one mile, and ftones of lefs fize to the diftance of
" three miles.   This eruption was accompanied by a
" great darknefs which continued many weeks.

  " Alphonfus Borelleús, a learned mathematician of
" Pifa, went into Sicily, while the fact was frefh, to
" view and furvey what Ætna had done ; and he fays,
" the quantity of matter thrown out at that time, up-
" on furvey, amounted to 93,838,750 cubical paces ;
" fo that had it been extended in length upon the fur-
" face of the earth, it would have reached farther than
" 93,000,000 of fuch paces, which is more than four
" times the circuit of the whole earth, taking 1000
" paces to a mile : 'tis true, all this matter was not
" liquid fire, but in part fand, ftone, gravel, &c. how-
" ever he computes 63,000,000 paces of this mat-
" ter were liquid fire, and formed a river, fome-
" times two miles broad, according to his computa-
" tion ; but according to the obfervation of others,
" who alfo viewed it, the torrent of fire was fix or fe-
" ven miles bioad, and fometimes ten or fifteen fa-
" thoms deep, and it forced its way into the fea near
" one mile, preferving itfelf alive in the midft of the
" waters.   He likewife obferves, that a ftone fifteen
                                                " feet

" feet long was flung out of the mouth of the pit
" to a mile diftance ; and when it fell, it came from
" fuch an height, and with fuch violence, that it bu-
" ried itfelf in the ground eight feet deep." See
Burnet's Sacred Theory, vol. ii. p. 82, 83.

42. Confiderable as the above eruptions may appear, a greater quantity of matter feems to have been
thrown out by a volcano in Peru, in the year 1600,
viz. " a fhower of afhes, fand, &c. covered all the
" land thirty leagues one way, and forty leagues an-
" other, round about Arequepa, from fix feet to eight
" or nine inches deep."* Whence it appears, that an
area of ground equal to 34,650 fquare miles was thus
covered.

43. " A mountain in Java, not far from the town
" of Panacura, in the year 1586, was fhattered to
" pieces by a violent eruption of glowing fulphur (tho'
" it had never burnt before) whereby 10,000 people
" perifhed in the under-land fields. It threw up large
" ftones, and caft them as far as Pancras." Varenius's Geog. vol. 1. p. 150.

Thus the fragments of the ftony *firata* are fpread
over the furface of the earth, to the diftance of many
miles fiom the craters of volcanos : and therefore, fince
fubterraneous explofions aie the only caufes, in Nature,

yet

* Dr. Hooke's Pofth. p. 304.

yet difcovered, whence fuch phenomena arife ; may we not thence conclude, that all fimilar appearances on the furface of the earth, are effects of the fame caufe ? notwithftanding there are no veftiges of ancient volcanos now remaining in many parts of the world where thefe fragments are fo fcattered about.

Were we to enumerate all the exifting volcanos in the different regions of the earth, together with thofe which have apparently been extinguifhed time immemorial ; and likewife the many inftances of new volcanos burfting forth, we fhould be apt to conclude, that fubterraneous fires either do or have heretofore exifted univerfally in the bowels of the earth.

We have therefore great reafon to prefume, from the analogy between the effects produced by fubterraneous fires, and the prefent ftate and condition of the earth, defcribed in chap. viii. that all the apparent confufion and diforder of the *ftrata*, are the undoubted effects of fubterraneous convulfions.

Yet it muft, however, be owned, that notwithftanding the effects of thefe *tremendous operations* of *Nature*, are, in many refpects, perfectly *analogous* to the *rude, romantic appearances* on the fuperficial parts of the earth : neverthelefs, when they are compared to thofe vaft eminences, the Alps, the Andes, &c. in point

of

of magnitude, the former feem to vanifh, or become too inconfiderable to ftand in competition with the latter.

Whence it appears, that fubterraneous convulfions weie much more violent in the early ages of the world, than they have been fince the commencement of hiftory : therefore, as the laws of Nature are conftant and immutable, it becomes neceffary to inquire why they operated with a greater degree of violence anterior to hiftoiy, than they have done within the laft period of two or three thoufand years. I fhall theiefoie endeavour to inveftigate this phenomenon in the enfuing chapter, and fhew, that it was a confequence neceffarily aiifing from the nature of things.

L   C H A P.

CHAP. XI.

On the Alterations produced by subterraneous Fires, on the superficial Parts of the Earth, anterior to History.

IN the preceding chapter we have enumerated some of the most considerable alterations which have happened to the superficial parts of the earth, since the commencement of history, in order to observe the analogy between those effects and the general state and condition of the terraqueous globe, with respect to its craggy rocks, mountains, vallies, &c. Whence it appears, that greater inequalities were produced in the early ages of the world, by subterraneous fires, than any we find upon record ; let us therefore endeavour to ascertain the truth of these conjectures in the following inquiry.

Those remote operations of Nature, I presume, have but lately engaged the attention of European philosophers, although it is so considerable a branch of natural history, and so essentially necessary to the investigation of many phenomena on the superficial and interior parts of the earth.

M. Con-

M. Condamine feems to be the firft naturalift who has taken this fubject into confideration, and at fo late a period as the year 1755. See his Tour to Italy.

Since that period the Honourable Sir William Hamilton, his Majefty's plenipotentiary at the court of Naples, has happily taken up the fubject, and carried his obfervations to a much greater length.

However, thofe of M Condamine I confider as very ingenious, and worthy of farther obfervation---

" All the mountains and hills about Naples," fays he,
" will be found, upon examination, to be huge heaps
" of matter, vomited out by volcanos which are now
" extinct, whofe eruptions, anterior to hiftory, feem to
" have formed the ports of Naples and Puzzoli. It is
" not in Naples alone, and its neighbourhood, that I
" have met with fuch like fubftances. As my eyes have
" been accuftomed to diftinguifh the different ema-
" nations of Vefuvius, and efpecially the lava, under
" its variety of afpects, I could trace it with eafe and
" certainty the whole way fiom Naples to Rome,
" even to the very gates, fometimes pure, and again
" combined with other fubftances.

" The whole infide of the mountain Fiafcati,
" where was Cicero's Tufculum; the chain of hills
" which extend from Frafcata to Grotta-Ferrata, Ca-

" ftel-

" ftel-Gondolfo, and even to the lake Albano ; a
" good part of the mountain Tivoli ; thofe of Ca-
" pravola, Viterbo, &c. confift of beds of calcined
" ftones, puie afhes, cinders, gravel, a fubftance like
" iron drofs, terra-cotta, and lava propeily fo called :
" in a word, fo like, in all refpects, to the compofi-
" tion of the foil of Portici, and to the materials
" which have iffued out of the fides of Vefuvius, un-
" der fuch a diverfity of forms, that the fight alone is
" fufficient to diftinguifh all thefe feveral fubftances.
" The afhes are manifeft, both from their colour and
" tafte.   It is impoffible foi any one who has atten-
" tively examined the productions of Vefuvius, not to
" be fatisfied of a peifect iefemblance between them
" and thofe he will meet with at eveiy ftep, in his
" way from Naples to Rome, fiom Rome to Viteibo,
" from Rome to Loretto, &c.

        " It then neceffaiily follows, that all this pait of
" Italy has been ruined by volcanos.   Thofe plains,
" now fo fmiling and feitile in olive-tiees, mulbeiiy-
" tiees, and vines, like the hills at prefent about Ve-
" fuvius, have like them been overfpiead with burning
" inundations, and bear, as they do, not only within,
" but on their fuiface, infallible maiks of fiery tor-
" rents, whofe waves are now fixed and confolidated,
                                " beaiing

" bearing teftimony of vaft ignitions, prior to all mo-
" numents of hiftory.

" When I fee, on an elevated plain, a circular ba-
" fon, furrounded with calcined rocks ; the verdure
" with which the neighbouring fields are covered, im-
" pofe not on me : I inftantly perceive the ruins of an
" ancient volcano, as 1 fhould perceive, beneath the
" fnow itfelf, the traces of an extinguifhed fire, on fee-
" ing an heap of cinders.

" If there be a breach in the circle, I ufually find out,
" by following the declivity of the ground, the traces
" of a rivulet, or the bed of a torrent, which feems as
" it were hollowed in the rock ; and this rock, when
" examined clofely, appears frequently to be nothing
" more than lava, properly fo called.

" If the circumference of the bafon has no breach,
" the rain and fpring waters which affemble there hav-
" ing no iffue, generally form a lake in the very
" mouth of the volcano.

" A few days after the fight of the lake Albano it-
" felf, (and the calcined matter with which its banks
" are powdered, left no room to doubt any longer of
" its origin.) I faw manifeftly the profound funnel or
" fhaft of an ancient volcano, in the mouth of which
" the waters had accumulated themfelves. Its erup-

" tion

" tion, of which hiftory makes no mention, muft have
" been anterior to the foundations of Rome, and even
" of Alba, from whence this lake has taken its name :
" a period amounting to near three thoufand years.

" At the fight of the traces of fire diffufed in the
" environs of the lakes of Borfello, de Rociglione, and
" Bracciano, on the road from Rome to Florence, I
" had formed the fame conjectures, before I had feen
" either Vefuvius, or the matter which it vomits forth.
" I pafs the fame judgment, by analogy, on the lake
" Perugia, and feveral others in the interior part of
" Italy, which I only know by the map.

" In fhort, I look upon the Appenines as a
" chain of volcanos, like that of the Cordeliers of
" Peru and Chily, which run from north to fouth,
" the whole length of South America, from the pro-
" vince of Quito to the Terra Magellanica.

" The courfe of the volcanos of the Cordeliers is
" interrupted , a great number of them are either ex-
" tinguifhed or fmothered, but feveral ftill remain ac-
" tually burning.   The old ones alfo frequently revive
" and fometimes new ones are kindled, even in the
" bottom of the fea.   Nor are their effects, on that
" account, lefs fatal.

                                          " A few

" A few years fince both Lima and Quito, two
" capital cities of Peru, became the victims of thofe
" two kinds of volcanos.

" The chain of the Appennines which divides the
" continent of Italy, in like manner from north to
" fouth, and extends as far as Sicily, prefents us ftill
" with a pretty great number of vifible fires under
" different forms.

" In Tufcany the exhalations of Firenzuolo, and
" the warm baths of Piza in the ecclefiaftical ftate,
" thofe of Viterbo, Norcia, Nocera, &c. in the
" kingdom of Naples, thofe of Ifchia, Solfataira, Ve-
" fuvius; in Sicily and the neighbouring ifles, Ætna,
" or Mount Gibel, with the volcanos of Lipari,
" Stromboli, &c. But other volcanos of the fame
" chain, having been quite extinguifhed fiom time
" immemoiial, have left only fome remains behind,
" which, though they may not always ftiike at firft
" fight, are not at all lefs diftinguifhable to attentive
" eyes.

" In fhort, the earthquakes which at various times
" have over-iun feveial of the cities of Italy and Si-
" cily; that which fwallowed up St. Euphemia in
" 1538; that which deftroyed Catana in 1693; that
" which opened the gulphs of Paleimo in 1718, and
" that

" that which over-run Syracufe, recall to my remem-
" brance the difafters of Valparaifo, Callao, Lima and
" Quito, in South America, and clofe the parallel be-
" tween the Cordeliers of Italy and thofe of Peru:
" the features of refemblance are but too ftriking.

" I do not affirm that all mountains are in the cafe
" of the Appennines; I could not obferve the fame
" appearances in that part of the Alps which I tra-
" veled over; but I have found the fame in Dauphiny,
" Provence, and feveral places where they were never
" looked upon as the effects of fire. It is not therefore
" in Italy alone that the veftiges of calcination and vitri-
" fication are to be met with, but alfo in places where
" volcanos have never been fuppofed to have exifted;
" France affords inflances, and poffibly moft coun-
" tries. My conjectures about the ancient volcanos
" of Italy, of which I find marks in all parts, and on
" the lava, which I difcovered even in places where
" I the leaft expected it, appear to me fo evident, that
" my only wonder was, they fhould be new. They
" were however looked upon as whims, in a country,
" where I ftill think, nothing more than the ufe of
" one's eyes is neceffary to produce the like, &c."

Thus far the obfervations of M Condamine, which
are happily confirmed by thofe of his excellency Sir
William

William Hamilton, who has alfo added many new and interefting obfervations on the ancient volcanos of Italy.

"It would require," fays he, "many yeais clofe "application to give a proper and truly philofophical "account of the volcanos in the neighbourhood of "Naples; but I am fure fuch an hiftory might be giv- "en, fupported by demonftration, as would deftroy "every fyftem hitherto upon the fubject.

"We have here an opportunity of feeing volcanos "in all their different ftates. I have been this fummer "in the ifland of Ifchia; it is about eighteen miles "round, and its whole bafe is lava. The great "mountain in it, near as high as Vefuvius, I am con- "vinced, was thrown up by degrees; and I have no "doubt in my own mind, but that the ifland itfelf "rofe out of the fea; in the fame manner as fome of "the Azores.

"I am of the fame opinion with refpect to mount "Vefuvius, and all the high grounds near Naples; "having not yet feen in any place, what can be cal- "led virgin earth.

"I had the pleafure of feeing a well funk at the "foot of Vefuvius, and clofe by the fea fide. At "twenty-five feet below the level of the fea, they

M   "came

" came to a *ftratum* of lava, and God knows how
" much deeper they might have ftill found other lavas.

" At the convent of the Dominican friars, called
" Madona del Areo, fome years ago, in finking a well,
" 100 feet deep, a lava was difcvered, and foon after
" another ; fo that in lefs than 300 feet deep, the
" lavas of four eruptions were found.

" From the fituation of this convent, it is clear,
" beyond a doubt, that thofe lavas proceeded from the
" mountain called Somma, as they are quite out of
" the reach of the exifting volcano.

" From thefe circumftances, and from the repeated
" obfervations that I have made in the neighbourhood
" of Vefuvius, I am fure no virgin foil is to be found
" there, but that all is compofed of different *ftrata* of
" erupted matter, even to a great depth below the
" level of the fea.

" In fhort, I have not any doubt in my own mind,
" but that this volcano took its rife from the bottom
" of the fea ; and as the whole plain between Vefu-
" vius and the mountains behind Caferta, which is beft
" part of Campania-Felice, is under its good foil com-
" pofed of burnt matter ; I imagine the fea to have
" wafhed the feet of thofe mountains, until the fub-
" terraneous fires began to operate, at a period cer-
" tainly of the moft remote antiquity.

" The

" The mountains at the back of Caferta are moftly
" a foit of limeftone, and therefore very different from
" thofe formed by fire; though Signor Van Vitelli, the
" celebrated architect, has affured me, that in cutting
" the famous aqueduct of Caferta through thofe moun-
" tains, he met with fome foils that had been evident-
" ly formed by fubterraneous fires."   Sir Wm. Hamilton's Obfervations on Vefuvius and Ætna.

Many other inftances might be added, to fhew that
the effects of volcanos, in the early ages of the world,
were much fuperior to thofe which have happened
within the laft period of two or three thoufand years :
which leads us to a further inquiry why greater effects
were produced in the early ages of the world, than
have been fince the commencement of hiftory.

L 2   CHAP.

C H A P. XII.

*Of subterraneous Fire, and its Effects, from the first
Increment of Heat to its full Maturity. Of the
Deluge. Of the Origin of Mountains, Continents,
&c. Of the Improbability of a second universal
Flood.*

THE inftances we find recorded of volcanos, and
their effects, leave no room to doubt the *existence*,
force, and *immensity* of fubterraneous fires ; not only
under the bottom of the ocean, but likewife under
mountains, continents, &c. in all parts of the world.

But from what principles they were generated, at
what diftance of time from the creation of the world,
or whether nearer to its center or to its furface, is perhaps not afcertainable, whilft the phenomena of fire
remain in fo much obfcurity : for, according to the celebrated chymift M. Macquer, " an accurate diftinc-
" tion has not yet been made between the phenomena
" of fire actually exifting as a principle in the compo-
" fition of bodies, and thofe which it exhibits when
" exifting feparately in its natural ftate : nor have pro-

3   " per

" per and diftinct appellations been affigned to it un-
" der thofe different circumftances :" * therefore, neither the *time*, the *place*, nor the *mode*, in which fubterraneous fire was generated, can be truly áfcertained.

However, this we know moft affuredly, that a certain degree of moifture and drynefs are productive of
fire in the vegetable and mineral kingdoms ; and likewife, that thofe fires are generated from the firft increment of heat, and gradually increafe to their full maturity.   Therefore, if we were allowed to reafon from
the analogy one part of nature bears to another, we
fhould conclude, that fubterraneous fire was generated
from the fame elementary principles, and alfo gradually
increafed to its full maturity.

Having premifed thefe matters, let us return to the
chaotic ftate of the earth, and endeavour to trace the
progreffive operations of fubterraneous fire, from its
firft increment of heat, and mark its effects on the incumbent *ftrata.*

1. If a certain degree of moifture and drynefs
were equally as neceffary to the production of fire in
the bowels of the earth as in the vegetable and mineral kingdoms, it feems to follow, that thofe parts of the
globe which firft began to confolidate, were alfo the
firft which began to generate fire : therefore as the central

* See Elements of Chymiftry, vol. i p. 7.

tral parts began to confolidate fooner than the more fuperficial, parts, (fee chap. v.) there is fome probability that they were the firft ignited.

2. It has alfo been obferved, (chap. v.) that as the earth began to confolidate by the union of fimilar particles, an univerfal famenefs prevailed either in the fame *ftratum*, or in the central part of the earth : whence it appears, that fubterraneous fire was generated univerfally in the fame point of time, either in the fame *ftratum* or in the central part of the earth, and gradually increafed to its full maturity.

3. All bodies expand with heat, and the force or power of that law is unlimited : therefore, as fubterraneous fire increafed, its expanfive force would gradually increafe, until it became equal to the incumbent weight. Gravity and expanfion being then equal, and the latter continuing to increafe, became fuperior to the former, and diftended the incumbent *ftrata*, as a bladder forcibly blown.

4. Now if this fire was furrounded by a fhell, or cruft of *equal thicknefs*, and of *equal denfity*, its *incumbent weight* muft have been *equal :* on the contrary, if the furrounding fhell or cruft were *unequally thick*, or *unequally denfe*, its incumbent weight muft have been unequal.

.5. Hence

5. Hence it appears, that as the primitive iſlands were uniform protuberances gradually aſcending from the deep, ſee chap. vi. the incumbent weight muſt have been unequal ; for as the ſpecific gravity of ſtone, ſand, or mud, is greater than that of water, the incumbent weight of the former muſt have been greater than that of the latter.

For example : Let plate VIII. repreſent a ſection of the antediluvian earth ; A B C, the primitive iſlands ; D D the bottom of the ocean ; and F F a *ſtratum* of ſubterraneous fire.

Now the incumbent weight, at A B C, being greater than at D D, the bottom of the ſea would conſequently aſcend, by the expanſive force of F F, ſooner than the iſlands A B C. The bottom of the ſea being thus elevated, the incumbent water would flow towards the leſs elevated parts to reſtore the equilibrium of its preſſure. See p. 63. § 25. Conſequently the iſland A B C, became more or leſs deluged, as the bottom of the ſea was more or leſs elevated ; and this effect muſt have been more or leſs univerſal, as the fire prevailed more or leſs univerſally, either in the ſame *ſtratum*, or in the central part of the earth. Therefore, ſince it appears, § 2. that ſubterraneous fire operated univerſally in the ſame *ſtratum*, with the ſame degree of force,

it

it appears much more probable, that the deluge prevailed univerfally over the earth, than partially ; and more efpecially when we confider the elevation of the antediluvian hills, according to chap. vi. But more of this hereafter.

But the tragical fcene endeth not with an univerfal flood, and the deftruction of terreftrial animals : for the expanfive force of fubterraneous fire, ftill increafing, became fuperior to the incumbent *weight* and *cohefion* of the *ftrata*, which were then burft, and opened a communication between the two oceans of melted matter and water.

The two elements coming thus into contact, the *latter* would be inftantaneoufly converted into fteam, and produce an explofion infinitely beyond all human conception ; for it is well known, that the expanfive force of water thus converted into fteam exceeds that of gunpowder in the proportion of fourteen thoufand to five hundred.*

The terraqueous globe being thus burft into millions of fragments, and from a caufe apparently feated

---

* The expanfive force of water converted into fteam, by different degrees of heat, has lately been inveftigated experimentally ; and I am informed the ingenious author intends to prefent his obfervations to the public.

nearer

nearer to its center than its furface, muft certainly be thrown into ftrange heaps of ruins : for the fragments of the *ftrata* thus blown up, could not poffibly fall together again into their primitive order and regularity : therefore an infinite number of fubterraneous caverns muft have been formed, probably many miles, or many hundreds of miles below the bottom of the antediluvian fea.

Now it is eafy to conceive, when a body of fuch an immenfe magnitude as the earth was thus reduced to an heap of ruins, that its *incumbent water* would immediately defcend into the caverns and interftices thereof ; and by approaching fo much nearer towards the center, than in its antediluvian ftate, much of the terreftrial furface would be left naked and expofed, with all its horrid gulphs, craggy rocks, mountains, and other diforderly appearances.

Thus the primitive ftate of the earth feems to have been totally metamorphofed by the firft convulfion of Nature, at the time of the deluge , its *ftrata* broken, and thrown into every poffible degree of confufion and diforder. Thus, thofe mighty eminences the Alps, the Andes, the Pyrenean mountains, &c. were brought from beneath the great deep---the fea retired from thofe vaft tracts of land, the continents----became fathom-

N   lefs,.

lefs; environed with craggy rocks, cliffs, and impending fhores; and its bottom fpread over with mountains
and vallies like the land.

It is further to be obferved of the horrid effects of
this convulfion----that as the primitive iflands were
more *ponderous* and *lefs elevated* than the bottom of
the fea, the former would more inftantaneoufly fubfide into the ocean of melted matter, than the latter :
therefore, in all probability, they became the bottom
of the poftdiluvian fea : and the bottom of the antediluvian fea being more elevated, was converted into
the poftdiluvian mountains, continents, &c. This conjecture is remarkably confirmed by the vaft number of
foffil fhells, and other marine *exuviæ*, found imbedded
near the tops of mountains, and the interior parts of
continents, far remote from the fea, in all parts of the
world hitherto explored.

The above phenomena have generally been afcribed
to the effects of an univerfal flood ; but we prefume
fuch conclufions were too haftily drawn : for it manifeftly appears, upon a more ftrict examination of the
various circumftances accompanying thefe marine bodies ; that they were actually generated, *lived*, and
died, in the very beds wherein they are found ; and
that thofe beds were originally the bottom of the
ocean,

ocean,* though now elevated several miles above its level. Thus we find a further agreement between natural phenomena and the laws of Nature.

Hence it appears, that mountains and continents were not primary productions of Nature ; but of a very diſtant period of time from the creation of the world.

It may, perhaps, be objected, that many of the above foſſil bodies are natives of very diſtant regions of the earth, and could not have exiſted in climates wherein they are found, according to the preſent conſtitution of Nature. Theſe objections will be conſidered in the following chapter.

To avoid prolixity, in the inveſtigation of the deluge, &c. many intereſting phenomena reſpecting earthquakes have been omitted : we ſhall, therefore, take this opportunity of introducing ſome of them, before we proceed to ſhew the improbability of a ſecond univerſal flood.

1. Previous to an eruption of Veſuvius, the ſea retires from its adjacent ſhores, and leaves its bottom dry, till the mountain is burſt open, when the water returns to its former boundary.

* See chap. vii

2. Before

2. Before volcanos burſt open the bottom of the ſea, the water riſes in thoſe places, conſiderably above its former level, runs in mountainous waves, towards the leſs elevated parts and deluges diſtant ſhores. See p. 63, § 25.

3. The earth is frequently burſt open many miles in length, and diſcharges ſuch vaſt quantities of water as to deluge the adjacent countries, of which we have had ſeveral inſtances, both in Europe and South America. In the year 1631, ſeveral towns were deſtroyed by an eruption of boiling water from Veſuvius ; and in the year 1755, an immenſe torrent of boiling water flowed from Ætna, a mile and a quarter broad, down to its baſe.   See Sir Wm. Hamilton's Obſervations on Veſuvius and Ætna, p. 82.

4. Eruptions are generally accompanied with thunder and lightning, and ſucceeded by inceſſant rains.

5. On the 1ſt of November 1755, the memorable æra of the earthquake at Liſbon, not only the ſea, but lakes and ponds were violently agitated all over Europe.   See Philoſ. Tranſ. vol. 79.

Moſt of theſe phenomena teſtify the immenſe force of ſteam generated by melted matter and water, in the bowels of the earth ; for, in the firſt inſtance, Mount Veſuvius and its adjacent ſhores being more elevated

by

by the fteams, than the bottom of the diftant fea ; the water retreats from the fhores towards the lefs elevated parts, and leaves its bottom dry. When the fteams find vent, by the eruption, the mountain fubfides to its former level, and the water returns to the fhore.

The fecond inftance fhews, that the bottom of the fea is more elevated than the land ; therefore the water retires, in mountainous waves, towards the lefs elevated parts, and overflows the coaft.

The third is not only a corroborating inftance, to fhew the expanfive foice of fteam ; but likewife coincides with the Mofaic defcription of the deluge, " *the* " *fountains of the great deep were broken up.*"

The fourth feems to have fome analogy to that dreadful event.

The fifth phenomenon feems to aiife fiom the fame caufe. When the *ftrata* incumbent on the melted matter aie elevated by the force of fteam , the impending roof is appaiently feparated from the liquid mafs ; and this feparation may be laterally extended to the diftance of many miles fiom the oiiginal fource of the fteam, according to its quantity, and degree of its expanfive foice.

Now if thefe conjectures aie true, the confequences thence aiifing aie manifeft. The *ftrata* immediately over

over the fteam fiift generated being more elevated than thofe in the act of feparation, the horizontal pofition of the earth's furface muft confequently be altered, fo as to pioduce an undulation of the water in lakes, ponds, &c. as in veffels fuddenly elevated on one fide more than on the other ; and thus continue in motion, alternately oveiflowing the oppofite banks, until the *momentum* acquired by the firft impulfe is gradually overcome.

That fteam is the principal agent whence thefe phenomena arife, I piefume will be readily granted by thofe who have caiefully attended to the Rev. Mr. Michell's obfeivations on the caufe of eaithquakes. Now, as one of the piopeities of fteam is condenfation by a fmall degiee of cold, the fame degiee of expanfive foice can only exift during the fame degiee of heat : therefoie the incumbent weight cannot become elevated to any gieatei diftance than fubterianeous fire is continued. This being granted, it feems to follow, tha as the wateis weie thus agitated on the 1ft of November 1755, through an extent of countiy not lefs than 3000 miles, theie muft have been one continued unintenupted mafs of melted mattei of the fame extent at leaft. And this idea feems to be conoboiated by thofe vaft explofions which were heaid in fome of the

3

Deiby-

Derbyſhire mines, about ten o'clock in the morning ſo fatal to Liſbon.   See Appendix.

The above examples ſerve to illuſtrate the powerful and extenſive effects of ſteam, produced by melted matter and water : truths well known to founders, particularly to thoſe converſant in caſting gold, ſilver, copper, braſs, and iron. " About ſixty years " ago, a melancholy accident happened from the caſt- " ing of braſs cannon, at Windmill-Hill, Moorfields, " where many ſpectators were aſſembled to ſee the me- " tal run into the moulds.   The heat of the metal " of the firſt gun drove ſo much damp into the mould " of the ſecond, which was near it, that as ſoon as the " metal was let into it, it blew up with the greateſt vi- " olence, tearing up the ground ſome feet deep, break- " ing down the furnace, untiling the houſe, killing " many people on the ſpot with the ſtreams of melted " metal," &c.   See Cramer's Art of Aſſaying Metals. Engliſh tranſlation, p. 323.

The inflammable vapour or damp, in mines, occaſions violent exploſions , but they are only momentary, as the firing of gunpowder.   On the contrary, thoſe from volcanos frequently continue many months, with great violence, which plainly ſhews that thoſe ſteams muſt be continually generating from the above cauſes.

Having

Having endeavoured to trace the progreſſive operations of ſubterraneous fire ; the cauſe of an univerſal flood ; the origin of mountains, continents, and other irregular appearances, on the ſurface and interior paits of the earth ; I purpoſe now to inquire into the improbability of a ſecond univerſal deluge ; and to ſhew why ſubterraneous convulſions produced more violent effects in the early ages of the world than they have done ſince the commencement of recoids.

It will readily be granted that the *ſtrata* had originally an *uniform, concentric arrangement* ; and likewife that they had acquired their greateſt degree of cohefion and firmneſs, previous to their being buiſt and thrown into heaps of confuſion : it is therefore evident that a much greater degiee of force was iequiſite to overcome the incumbent weight and cohefion of the *ſtrata*, in that *firm, uniform ſtate*, than can be requiſite to ſepaiate the fiactuied paits thereof ; conſequently, the fame degiee of power can never be accumulated, whilſt ſo many fiſſuies and volcanos daily give vent to the expanſive vapouis, and thereby counteract their violence.

Now as the expanſive force of ſubteiraneous ſteams in the poſtdiluvian world is fo much infciior to thoſe in the antediluvian ſtate of nature, and the mountains

I   of

of the former fo much fuperior to the hills of the latter ; the prefumption is great, that the earth can never
be deluged a fecond time from the fame caufe ; nor its
ftrata fuffer the fame degree of violence.

But after all our refearches into thefe vaft operations
of Nature, the magnitude of the earth fo much exceeds
the bounds of human conception, that we can form no
adequate idea of its bulk, nor of the relation the mountains, and other inequalities, bear to its diameter :
therefore, let us reduce it to fuch a fcale as we can di-
ftinctly view and comprehend.

Now as the earth is nearly 8000 miles diameter, it
may be fufficiently accurate for our purpofe, to reduce
it to a fcale of 80 inches ; fince one inch will then
bear the fame proportion to a globe of 80 inches diameter, as 100 miles does to the diameter of the earth.

As one-tenth of an inch is to a globe 80 inches diameter : fo is a mountain 10 miles perpendicular height,
to the earth.

Again, as one-hundredth part of an inch is to a
globe of 80 inches, diameter : fo is a mountain one
mile perpendicular height to the earth.

And as the thicknefs of a human hair is nearly equal
to one four-hundredth part of an inch, it will nearly
bear the fame proportion to a globe 80 inches dia-

meter,

meter, as a mountain one-fourth of a mile perpendicular height does to the earth.

Thefe relations being duly confidered, we fhall be enabled to compare the elevation of the antediluvian hills with the poftdiluvian mountains. Some of the latter we know, from geometrical and barometrical menfuration are upwaids of three geometrical miles, 18,756 feet, above the level of the fea. [See Ulloa's Voyage, vol. i. p. 442.] Whereas we cannot fuppofe the former were more than 50 or 100 feet perpendicular height above it ; fince it appears, chap. vi. that they were formed by the action of the tides, as fand-banks are formed in the fea.

Now the inequalities on the earth's furface, before and after the flood, being thus compared, they affoid fome idea of the gieat alterations which the fuperficial part of the earth underwent at the time of the deluge ; and of the impoffibility of a fecond univerfal flood arifing from the fame caufe in any future age.

It remains now to inquire what effects were produced in the temperature of the air and feafons of the year, in confequence of this ftupendous convulfion of Nature.

P. S.

P. S. As the diftenfion of the *ftrata*, obferved in the
former part of this chapter, may appear highly improbable to fome readers, I take this opportunity of recit-
ing the reverend Mr. Michell's obfervations on the elafticity and compreffibility of ftone, &c. mentioned in his
excellent Treatife on Earthquakes, note, p. 34, as follows : " The compreffibility and elafticity of the earth
" are qualities which do not fhew themfelves in any
" great degree in common inftances, and therefore are
" not commonly attended to. On this account it is
" that few people are aware of the great extent of
" them, or the effects that may arife from them, where
" exceeding large quantities of matter are concerned,
" and where the compreffive force is immenfely great.
" The compreffibility and elafticity of the earth may
" be collected, in fome meafure, from the vibration of
" the walls of houfes, occafioned by the paffing of car-
" riages in the ftreets next to them. Another in-
" ftance, to the fame purpofe, may be taken from the
" vibration of fteeples, occafioned by the ringing of
" bells, or by gufts of wind : not only fpires are mo-
" ved very confiderably by this means, but even ftrong
" towers will fometimes be made to vibrate feveral
" inches, without any disjointing of the mortar, or
" rubbing the ftones againft one another. Now, it is
O 2 " manifeft,

" manifeſt, that this could not happen, without a
" conſiderable degree of compreſſibility and elaſticity
" in the materials of which they are compoſed."

Now, if ſo ſhort a length of ſtone as that of a ſtee-
ple, viſibly bends, by ſo ſmall a degree of force as the
ringing of bells, or a blaſt of wind , may we not conclude, that the *ſtrata*, in the primitive ſtate of the
earth, might become conſiderably diſtended, by an unlimited force [§ 3.] and therefore occaſion an univerſal deluge, according to the preceding concluſion,
p. 87, 88.   Since it appears that if a globe 80 inches
diameter only, ſuffered a degree of expanſion equal to
the thickneſs of a human hair ; the ſame degree of
heat, by analogy, would have raiſed the bottom of the
ocean one fourth of a mile ; which is above four times
higher than the primitive iſlands were ſuppoſed to have
been elevated above the ſurface of the ſea.

C H A P.

CHAP. XIII.

Of the Temperature of the Air, and Seasons of the Year, arising from the Production of Mountains and Continents at the Time of the Deluge.

IN the preceding chapter, we have endeavoured to prove *one* universal deluge; the improbability of a second; and to shew that mountains and continents were not *primary* productions of Nature, but of a very distant period of time from the creation of the world: a time when the *strata had acquired their greatest degree of cohesion and firmness,* and when the *marine shells* included in them were *totally changed* to a *stony substance.*

Let us therefore inquire what effects those great alterations on the superficial parts of the earth, occasioned in the temperature of the air, and seasons of the year, after the flood; when the altitude of the mountains was apparently 187 times higher than the hills in the antediluvian world.

This

This inquiry, happily dependeth on such phenomena as are commonly known though not afcertained with fo much accuracy in the different parts of the world, as the importance of the fubject requires.

1. It is generally obferved, that the interior parts of continents are fubject to greater extremes of heat and cold, than the exterior, or the coafts of the fea. Firft, fiom the continuance of *froft* and *fnow*, in the former, at a time when it will not lie on or near the coaft of the latter. Secondly, from the plants and fruits of the earth being burnt up within land, when there is an agreeable verduie on the fhore.

2. Hence Cornwall, being a peninfula, is lefs fubject to extremes of heat and cold, and to fudden tranfitions fiom one extreme to another, than the central parts of England : " vegetables flourfh all winter in the for-
" mer, which can only be preferved in the latter by
" artificial means : nor have they feldom any fioft till
" after Chriftmas, but a tempeiate aii, and an exceed-
" ing fine verdure on the ground ; their fpring feafons
" are indeed colder, and laft longer than in the central
" parts of England." See Dr. Boilace's Nat. Hift. of Cornwall.

3. " The temperature of the air in Norway diffeis
" more than a ftranger could well imagine in the fame
　　　　　　　　　　　　　　　　　" parallel

" parallel of latitude ; for on the eaft fide of Norway
" the winter's cold generally fets in about the middle
" of October, and continues to the middle of April ;
" the waters are frozen to a thick ice, and the moun--
" tains and vallies are covered with fnow.

4. " Yet when the winter rages with fo much fe-
" verity on the eaftern fide of Norway, the lakes and
" bays are open on the weftern fide, though in the fame
" parallel of latitude ; the air, indeed, is mifty and
" cloudy, but froft is feldom known to laft longer than
" a fortnight or three weeks.

5. " In the center of Germany, which is 200 leagues
" nearer the line, winters are more fevere than in the
" diocefs of Bergin, where the inhabitants often won-
" der to read in the public papers, of froft and fnow in
" Poland and Germany, when they have no fuch wea-
" ther there.

6. " The harbours of Amfterdam, Hamburgh, Co-
" penhagen and Lubeck, are frozen ten times oftener
" than the harbour of Bergin ; and when the harbour
" of Bergin is frozen, the Seine at Paris is generally in
" the fame condition.

7. " It feldom happens that the bays and creeks are
" frozen over in Norway, except thofe that run far up
" the country.   In the other parts of the weftern coaft,

2   " hard

" hard winters, or lafting frofts, are feldom heard of."
See Pontop. Nat. Hift. Norway.

8. " It is well known to all who fail northward, as
" far as lat. 77. that the coafts are frozen up many
" leagues, when the open fea is not fo ; no not even
" under the pole."

9. " Some years fince, a company of merchants at
" Amfterdam, who advanced 100 leagues above No-
" va Zembla, towards the eaft, difcovered a fea free
" fiom ice, and very convenient for navigation."
Lowthorp's Abridg. Phil. Tranf. vol. iii. p. 611.

10. " And we are well affuied, by the teftimony of
" Capt. Baffin, that the noithern parts of Greenland
" are lefs incumbeied with ice than the fouthern ;
" and that he found no ice in Baffin's Bay, though in
" lat. 74 ; and, as he advanced ftill further north, he
" found the air moie foft and tempeiate ; veiy diffe-
" ient fiom what he had felt in Davis's Straights, and
" on the fouth of Greenland."

11. " And it appeais, in the journals of Frederick
" Martin of Hamburgh, a man of good credit, that
" when Spitfbergen is doubled three or four degrees,
" to the north, no more ice is to be fcen."

12. " Capt. Wood likewife obferves, in a paper
" which he publifhed before he performed his voyage,

" that

" that two Dutch fhips had proceeded northward,
" as far as latitude 89°, and there found the fea free
" from ice, and of an unfathomable depth ; as ap-
" pears by four of their journals, which though fepa-
" rately kept, concur in thofe circumftances."

12. " Captain Wood farther adds, that a Dutch-
" man of great veracity had affured him, that he had
" paffed even under the pole, and found the weather
" as warm as at Amfterdam."*

13. Other navigators have alfo obferved, that the
weather was warm in lat. 88° north, and the fea perfectly free from ice, and rolling like the Bay of Bif-
cay.†

14. The fame author mentions another fhip having failed within half a degree of the pole ,‡ with many other interefting accounts of navigators having advanced to high latitudes ; infomuch that no doubt can
remain of the high feas under the pole being open, at
all times, and fit for navigation, though much incum-
bered with ice in lower latitudes.   The caufe of thefe
phenomena will be confidered in its due place.

---

* Univerfal Muf. Dec. 1776, p 565
  † See the Hon. Daines Barington's Obfervations on the Probability
of reaching the North Pole, p. 11.
  ‡ Ibid. p. 21.

15. The

15. The continent of North America, we are told, is subject to great extremes of heat and cold, and to sudden transitions from one extreme to another.

16. That in South Carolina, though situate almost twenty degrees more south than London, frost is sometimes very intense ; at others they have a degree of heat equal to 100° Fahrenheit's scale.

17. " At Cape Henry, lat. 36° 30' north, the tem-
" perature of the air and seasons are much govern-
" ed by the winds in Virginia, both as to heat and
" cold, moisture and dryness, the variations of which
" are very remarkable ; there being often great and
" sudden changes.   The north and north-west winds
" are very nitrous and piercing, cold and clear, or else
" stormy ; the south-east and south, hazy and sultry
" hot.   Their winter is a fine clear air, mild and dry,
" which renders it very pleasant ; their frosts are short,
" but sometimes so very sharp, as to freeze the ri-
" vers over, though three miles broad ; nay, even
" the Potomack river, where it is near nine miles,
" broad."*

18. We are also told, that their lakes and rivers are generally frozen over early in the winter, and remain in the same state till late in the spring, though situate

* Lowth. Abr. Phil. Transf. vol. iii. p. 576.

many

many degrees more fouth than the Land's-end of England, and that at Quebec the mercury will frequently mark 100° at one time and 40° or 50° below the freezing point at another.

19. In Maryland the temperature of the air has been truly afcertained by Fahrenheit's thermometer. The following table fhews the refult of four years obfervations, *viz.* 1754, 1755, 1756, 1757. See Philof. Tranf. vol. li. p. 62, 82. To which is added a comparative view of the climate of London, for the fame years; fhewing the greateft degree of heat and cold in each month.*

The firft column contains the months; the fecond, marked H, fhews the higheft ftate of the mercury; L, the loweft; and V, the variation in each month. Foi example: London, January 1754, the higheft ftate of the mercury was 48°, the loweft 25°, the variation 23°; Maryland, 61° the higheft, 21° the loweft, and 40° the variation.

* See Gentleman's Magazine for the above years.

P 2

LONDON.

Mon.	LONDON Lat 51° 30'												MARYLAND. Lat. 39°											
	1754			1755			1756			1757			1754			1755			1756			1757		
	H	L	V	H	L	V	H	L	V	H	L	V	H	L	V	H	L	V	H	L	V	H	L	V
Jan	48	25	23	45	27	18	49	39	10	44	28	16	61	21	40	69	23	46	73	15	58	65	10	55
Feb.	48	25	23	44	31	13	50	32	18	52	31	21	61	10	51	64	14	50	70	27	43	67	8	59
Mar	46	29	17	51	32	19	54	35	19	54	33	21	71	27	44	79	24	55	-	-	-	65	30	35
Apr	54	32	21	65	42	23	53	32	21	61	30	31	73	42	31	80	40	40	83	29	54	65	30	35
May	-	-	-	64	45	19	64	37	27	64	45	19	85	45	40	87	47	40	81	48	33	88	48	40
June	-	-	-	77	61	16	70	48	22	67	56	11	87	56	31	93	70	20	86	44	42	80	72	18
July	-	-		70	55	15	68	51	17	77	59	18	87	61	26	93	60	33	93	69	24	90	64	26
Aug	-	-	-	66	52	14	65	-	-	76	54	22	88	62	26	90	61	29	93	68	25	90	67	23
Sept	64	43	21	67	48	21	64	50	14	61	53	8	80	73	7	93	45	48	92	60	32	88	47	41
Oct	56	39	17	65	41	24	62	30	32	56	42	14	80	34	46	75	36	39	90	29	61	67	43	24
Nov	49	27	22	55	28	27	54	31	23	55	38	17	67	23	44	65	20	46	73	27	46	65	33	32
Dec	-	-	-	50	34	16	51	31	20	51	35	16	60	23	37	71	15	56	63	13	50	68	28	40

By thus comparing the climate of London with that
of Maryland, it appears, that the latter is fubject to
much greater extremes of heat and cold than the former.*

The

* Although Fahrenheit's thermometer is generally known, it may
not be improper to name the relative degrees of heat and cold refer-
red to in the above table. For example 32° marks the firft increment

The following table is a farther teftimony, that the continent of America is not only fubject to great extremes of heat and cold ; but likewife to great and fudden changes from one extreme to another.

The firft column contains the year, month, and day. Thofe N° 1, 2, 3, fhew the ftate of the mercury, 1. morning, 2. noon, and 3. evening. The column D, fhews the variation of temperature each day ; M, the monthly variation.

Thofe numbers marked thus — denote the number of degrees below o. For example : January 3, the number —24, fignifies that the mercury was 24° below o, or 56° below the freezing point.†

ment of freezing ; 48° the temperature of common fpring water ; 68° that of Matlock Bath , 82° Buxton Bath , 96° vital heat ; 114° King's Bath, at Bath , 212° the heat of boiling water , and likewife, that cold increafes in the fame proportion below the freezing point.

† Notwithftanding the fuperiority of Fahrenheit's fcale, it is much to be wifhed the freezing point had been marked o, as it would have fimplified the mode of regiftering the obfervations For inftance on the 6th of January in the morning, the mercury marked —29° below o, in the evening 35° above o, which fhews a variation in the temperature of the air, equal to 64° for 29 + 35 = 64 , therefore, by means of a fcale afcending and defcending from the freezing point, 64° would exprefs the degree of cold, and avoid the above numerical operation.

Obfer-

OBSERVATIONS *on the Temperature of the Air, at Prince of Wa'es Fort, on the north west coast of Hudson's Bay, in Lat. 58° 47' N. in the Years 1768 and 1769, by Mr.* William Wales *and Mr.* Joseph Dymond.

1768	1	2	3	D	M	1769	1	2	3	D	M	1769	1	2	3	D	M
Sept 10	41	41	41	0		Jan 3	—24	—16		8		May 3	45	32	37	13	
14	45	41	38	7		6	—29	31	35	64		6	50	35	39	15	
16	37	34		3		9	—19	—21	—30	11		9	49	45	26	23	
18	38	33		5		12	—28	—15	—17	13		12	23	24	22	2	
20	45	38		7	32	15	—21	—28	—31	10	71	15	40	27	32	13	
22	60	63	65	5		18	—32	—36	—30	6		18	54	32	44	22	32
24	54	50	46	8		21	—29	—36	—36	7		21	48	40	36	12	
28	46	46	44	2		24	—28	—31	—19	12		24	43	7	33	14	
30	47	50	35	15		27	—20	—31	—34	14		27	28	30	34	14	
												30	49	34	37	15	
Oct 3	36	34	29	7		Feb. 2	—1	—21	—30	29		June 3	60	42		18	
6	35	34	29	5		4	0	—19	—20	20		6	45	36	38	9	
9	35	37	34	3		6	—16	—23	—24	8		9	50	44	40	10	
12	32	31	33	2		9	15	12	12	3		12	41	39	40	2	
15	36	31	17	19	24	12	—3	—21	—26	29	52	15	46	41		5	28
18	33	32	32	1		15	3	—2	—11	14		18	50	44	35	15	
21	36	36	27	9		18	—4	—19	—18	15		21	63	57	41	22	
24	20	21	13	8		21	6	—20	—32	38		24	49	57	61	12	
27	28	27	14	14		24	—10	—29	—37	27		27	60	50	55	10	
30	22	18	20	4		28	—9	—12	—30	21		30	60	49	44	16	
Nov 3	32	24	18	14		Mar. 3	—13	—15	—30	17		July 3	76	80	74	6	
6	5	—10	—7	15		6	—19	—30	—41	22		6	54	46	45	8	
9	—3	3	4	7		9	—11	—11	6	17		9	51	50	61	11	
12	15	12	18	6		12	0	—5	—23	23		12	8c	48	52	33	
15	3	6	—5	11		15	—16	—21	—25	9	81	15	55	50	49	6	
18	—7	—14	—15	8	48	18	1	1	7	6		18	60	52	52	14	39
21	10	7	3	7		21	4	—8	—11	15		21	58	62	54	8	
24	7	1	—7	14		24	—5	—21	—23	18		24	64	59	56	8	
27	—15	—16	—16	1		27	40	24	11	29		27	59	63		6	
30	—10	—9	4	14		30	20	7	8	13		30	65	65	54	11	
Dec. 3	—6	—10	—17	11		April 3	7	7	—12	19		Aug. 3	50	64	48	6	
6	—16	—22	—26	10		6	20	—2	0	22		6	68	54	52	16	
9	—9	—13	—20	11		9	33	22	11	22		9	60	52	58	8	
12	—39	—39	—22	17		12	19	15	12	7		12	61	53	52	9	
15	—23	—27	—15	12		15	20	9	5	24	68	15	56	57	48	9	24
18	—8	—10	—16	8	65	18	34	26	20	14		18	40	43	41	6	
21	14	17	13	4		21	38	17	20	21		21	57	51			
24	17	26	—24	50		24	36	26	26	10		24	51	48		3	
27	11	15	—6	21		27	48	56	34	22		27	53	49	44	9	
30	6	—12	—18	23		30	36	29	32	7		30					

The preceding obfervations evidently fhew that the continent of North America is fubject to much *greater extremes* of *heat* and *cold* than England ; and likewife to more fudden tranfitions from one extreme to another : therefore, let us endeavour to compar the temperature of the air in Great Britain with that in iflands of lefs magnitude, and thofe with the temperature of the air at fea.

1. It is well known, that in the fouth-weft parts of Ireland, myrtles grow in common with other fhrubs, and that they even arrive to the amazing height of ten or twelve feet; though in moft parts of England they are only preferved by art, and perhaps, in no part of it, flourifh with the fame degree of luxuriancy : whence it appears, that the climate of Ireland is more temperate than that of England.

2. The Orkneys, we are told, are more fubject to rain than fnow or froft, which do not continue fo long as in other parts of Scotland.

3. In Farro Ifland, lat. 62° north, froft feldom continues longer than a month, and is withal fo moderate, that ice is never feen in an open bay ; nor are fheep or oxen ever brought under cover.

4. Madeira, fituate lat. 32° north, is not fubject to greater degrees of heat than England.

5. In

5. In Goree, lat. 15° north, they breathe a cool and temperate air, almoſt the whole year round, being continually refreſhed by land and ſea breezes.*

6. St. Helena, ſituate lat. 16° ſouth, is alſo extremely temperate, as appears by the obſervations of Dr. Maſkelyne, in the year 1761.†

Obſervations on the Temperature of the Air at ST. HELENA, 1761.

April				May		
	25	73°		1	72°
	26	73		2	72
	27	73		3	71
	28	73		4	71
	29	73		5	70
	30	72		6	70
				7	72
				8	72

7. And according to the obſervations of our late navigators, moſt of the iſlands in the ſouthern hemiſpheie, enjoy a degree of *temperature* and *fertility* much ſuperior to the *climate* of *England*.

Though it appears from various circumſtances, that iſlands of leſs magnitude than Great Britain are leſs

* Adenſon's Voyage, p. 104.
† Philoſ. Tranſ. p. 440.

subject to extremes of *heat* and *cold* ; yet the phenomenon of *land* and *fea* breezes, which generally accompany thofe within or near the tropicks, feems to fhew that they are fubject to greater tranfitions from heat to cold, than the atmofphere at fea : therefore, fince the temperature of the air on iflands has not been generally afcertained, it becomes neceffary to inveftigate the caufe of thofe alteinate breezes from *fea* and *land*, as the only teftimony to prove that the temperature of the former is more equable than the latter. The phenomenon is as follows :

1. In the middle, or hotteft part of the day, the fea breeze blows towards the land, in every poffible direction.

2. In the middle, or coldeft part of the night, the land breeze blows towards the fea, in every poffible direction, and thus they alternately fucceed each othei, as conftantly as night and day.

This extiaordinary phenomenon feems to aiife from the following unalterable laws of Nature : namely, thofe pioperties of the air by which it is fubject to rarefaction by heat and condenfation by cold ; and in part to the iflands being fituate within the toirid zone, wheie days and nights are nearly of equal length, at all times of the year.

Q

Now

Now it is a truth commonly known, that the fun's heat operates more powerfully on the furface of land than on the furface of water ; for the former not being a conductor of heat, it confequently accumulates upon its furface to a confiderable degree, more than on the furface of water ; therefore rarefies the incumbent air, more than the atmofphere at fea : for water being a conductor of heat, it becomes more equally diffufed throughout its whole mafs ; by this means the equilibrium of preffure between the two atmofpheres is deftroyed : therefore as the land atmofphere is rendered fpecifically lighter than the air at fea, the former afcends by the fuperior weight of the latter : therefore the fea breeze blows towards the land in every poffible direction. When night approaches, the fun's heat abates, until the land atmofphere becomes equally denfe with that at fea. The equilibrium of preffure being thus reftored, the fea breeze totally ceafes. Cold increafing by the abfence of the fun, and its fudden departure below the horizon, accumulates on the furface of the iflands, and condenfes their incumbent atmofpheres more than that at fea : for water being alfo a conductor of cold, it becomes equally diffufed throughout its whole mafs, and cannot accumulate as on the

fur-

furface of the land.* The land atmofphere being thus rendered fpecifically heavier than the air at fea, continually defcends, by its fuperior weight, and blows in all directions towards the fea , till the fun returns, and reftores the two atmofpheres to an equal denfity. The air then becomes ftagnant, and remains in a quiefcent ftate, till it is again rarified by the accumulation of heat, as before.

* That the fea has a property of conducting or diffufing heat and cold throughout its whole mafs, plainly appears from the experiments lately made on its temperature by Mr Bayley, on board his majefty's floop Adventure, on her late voyage towards the fouth.† The refult was as follows :

1772, Aug. 27	External air - -	72°¼
	The fea near its furface -	70°
	At the depth of 80 fathoms	68°
Dec. 27.	External air - -	31°¼
	The fea near its furface -	32°
	At the depth of 160 fathoms	33¼
1773, Aug. 28.	External air - -	64
	The fea near its furface -	59
	At the depth of 140 fathoms	56½

Hence the fea becomes the great regulator in the temperature of climates.

That land is not a conductor of heat and cold appears from the uniform temperature of fprings near the furface of the earth for water contained in wells not more than ten or twenty yards deep, varies nothing in its temperature, winter nor fummer being conftantly about 48° On the contrary, the fea conforms as above to the temperature of the atmofphere

† See the Aftronomical Obfervations, publifhed by Mr. Wales, p. 206, 208, 10

Thus

Thus by an alternate rarefaction and condenfation of the air at land, and an uniform temperature of the air at fea, the land and fea breezes fucceed each other with as much regularity as night and day.

Such are the apparent caufes of the land and fea breezes which accompany the iflands fituate within the torrid zone. Whence it appears that the temperature of the air at fea, is more conftant and uniform than upon iflands; and this conclufion is abundantly confirmed. by the obfervations contained in the following table..

Observations on the Temperature of the Air at Sea, on board his Majesty's Sloop Adventure, in her late Voyage on Discoveries towards the South by Mr William Bayley. The First Column contains the Year, Month, and Day The second Column shews the Latitude. The Columns 1, 2, 3, shew the Number of Observations each Day. D, the Variation of Heat and Cold each Day.

1772	Lat N.	1	2	3	D	1772	Lat S.	1	2	3	D	1773	Lat S	1	2	3	D
July 17	46	26	67	68	66	2	Nov 20	- -	-	-	-	-	Mar. 3	46 18	53	53	52	1
18	46	46	68	69	65	4	21	- -	-	-	-	-	6	43 57	53	52	51	2
19	45	20	65	64	65	1	22	33	55	-60	-	-	9	43 46	55	57	54	3
20	43	56	65	67	64	3	23	34	34	-65	-	-	Adventure Bay					
22	43	37	65	66	65	1	24	35	20	-63	-	-	12		57	58	52	6
24	40	3	66	67	67	1	25	37	14	-65	62	1	15	43 20	56	56	51	5
26	35	31	70	72	69	3	26	39	0	62	69	60	18	40 22	53	54	52	2
28	32	48	72	74	73	2	27	40	1	51	52	53	21	39 16	58	59	57	2
— Madeira.						28	40	55	53	59	52	24	38 58	57	58	52	5
30	- -	73	76	74	3	29	42	8	52	52	53	27	40 14	6	61	60	1
31	32	33	74	75	74	1	30	42	26	52	55	52	30	41 14	62	62	64	2
Aug 3	29	43	72	73	72	1	Dec. 3	44	27	47	48	46	April 3	40 40	62	63	60	3
6	26	6	73	73	72	1	6	48	23	36	36	35	6	41 4	63	61	57	6
9	0	28	74	75	74	1	9	49	46	33	34	35	Q Charlotte's Sound.					
12	15	7	77	79	78	2	12			32	34	32	9	- -	45	61	55	7
15	13	48	79	81	79	2	15	55	2	28	31	30	12	- -	54	62	56	8
18	11	25	77	81	77	4	18	54	59	31	31	30	15	- -	52	57	54	5
21	8	41	79	78	77	2	21	54	7	32	34	31	18	- -	-	-	-	
24	6	24	79	79	78	1	24	56	29	32	34	32	21	- -	53	59	59	6
27	4	13	78	78	78	0	27	58	21	32	35	32	24	- -	49	54	50	5
30	2	40	78	78	78	1	30	59	22	32	34	32	27	- -	44	57	54	13
31	2	40	78	78	78	0	31	59	55	0	-3	32	30	- -	50	54	51	
Sept 3	1	1	77	77	77	0	1773 Jan 3	59	23	31	32	31	May 1	- -	56	59	54	5
6	0	36	77	77	76	1	6	59	59	35	33	35	3	- -	47	57	45	1
Latitude South						9	61	36	2	35	33	6	- -	48	54	55	7
9	0	50	75	76	75	1	12	64	14	33	35	32	9	- -	57	58	51	
12	4	10	73	75	72	3	15	63	35	34	37	33	12	- -	54	52	49	5
15	8	10	73	75	72	3	18	65	58	33	34	33	15	- -	47	58	5	11
18	12	26	72	71	73	2	21	62	45	33	3	34	18	- -	52	5	47	11
21	17	9	73	73	72	1	24	58	24	4	35	3	21	- -	54	57	44	13
24	21	30	72	72	71	1	27	56	30	33	35	33	24	- -	19	51	49	3
27	24	40	70	71	70	2	30	51	31	39	39	34	27	- -	47	5	49	10
30	26	58	69	70	71	2							30	- -	59	59	52	7
Oct 3	28	4	66	66	64	2	Feb 3	49	15	44	44	43	June 1	- -	56	56	50	6
6	29	4	59	61	58	3	6	48	53	47	45	43	3	- -	53	58	51	7
9	33	52	59	59	57	2	9	50	17	43	43	41	6	- -	52	56	17	9
12	34	46	57	65	58	8	12	50	41	38	40	37	9	47 50	55	52	48	7
15	35	33	59	63	57	6	15	52	13	37	38	39	12	45 45	51	54	17	5
18	34	3	55	57	53	4	18	52	52	37	40	37	15	46 45	54	49	47	7
21	35	31	57	9	55	4	21	52	13	40	41	38	18	45 50	49	49	17	2
24	36	39	55	57	57	5	24	52	7	40	43	41	21	44 17	50	51	50	1
27	33	47	57	61	60	4	26	51	18	43	44	44	24	43 4	47	57	19	5
30	33	55	56				27	50	47	45	43	45	27	42 23	52	5	51	
Cape of Good Hope						28	50	21	43	43	44	30	43	51	52	50	

According to the preceding obfervations, the burning heats of the torrid zone, and the intenfe cold in the fiigid zone, are not altogether owing to their refpective fituations, but rathei to the different quantities of land. May we not therefore conclude, that if the terraqueous globe was univerfally covered with water, as in its piimitive ftate, that the temperature of the air, would yet be moie univeifally equable fiom pole to pole ; infomuch that froft and fnow could have no exiftence on the face of the earth ? For the high feas being open at all times, and not frozen at all, is appaiently owing to its being a part of the great Pacific Ocean, and the intenfe cold in lower latitudes, to the near approach of the two continents.

Now fince it appeais that extremes of heat and cold are confequences neceffarily arifing from mountains and continents : it evidently follows that they only commenced with the gieat alteiations wrought on the fupeificial parts of the eaith at the time of the deluge. Whence it appears, that the antediluvian ftate of Natuie was moie univerfally adapted to animal and vegetable life, than the poftdiluvian ftate of it. It is theiefore reafonable to fuppofe, that it was more univerfally inhabited by eveiy fpecies of the animal and vegetable cieation ; which I fhall endeavour to prove in the following chapter.

C H A P.

CHAP. XIV.

On the Temperature of the Air, and Seasons in the Antediluvian World. Of its being more universally habitable than the Postdiluvian World. Some Inquiry into the Cause of animal and vegetable Exuviæ being found remote from their native Climates.

HAVING enumerated many instances in the preceding chapter, to shew, that the burning heats of summer, and the severities of winter, commenced with the production of mountains and continents at the time of the deluge ; it becomes necessary now to enquire into the temperature of the *air* and *seasons* of the *antediluvian world*.

According to the chapters v. and vii. the terraqueous globe was originally covered with water, and its primitive islands raised from beneath the deep by the undulation of its tides, as sand banks are raised in the sea : whence it is presumed, they were of little extent or elevation, compared to the mountains and continents in the postdiluvian world.

3 Now

Now since it appears from the preceding obfervations, chapter xiii. that the burning heats in the torrid zone, and the intenfe cold in the frigid zone, are
not wholly owing to their refpective fituations or diftance from the line ; but principally to thofe vaft
tracts of land the continents : may we not therefore
conclude, that as the magnitude of the primitive
iflands was fo much inferior to that of the continents,
that the temperature of the air and feafons of the
former, were much lefs fubject to extremes of heat
and cold than the latter.

Such being the ftate of the antediluvian world, it
feems to follow, that its different regions were univerfally habitable; and therefore were inhabited by a
much greater variety of animals and vegetables, than
can now be fuppofed to exift in them according to the
prefent conftitution of Nature.

This being granted, it feems to unfold that wonderful phenomenon of foffil fhells, and other *exuviæ* of
marine animals and vegetables being found imbedded in
the earth, fo extremely remote from their native climates , and oftentimes depofited with as much order
as beds of living fhell-fifh are in the fea. See chap.
VII. p. 44.

2   Natural

Natural phenomena thus coinciding with the refult of phyfical reafoning, is a farther teftimony that the temperature of the air and feafons in the antediluvian world, were more univerfally adapted to animal and vegetable life, than the prefent conftitution of the atmofphere ; and likewife that its different regions were inhabited by a much greater variety of fpecies than they are at prefent.

The antediluvian world being thus univerfally inhabited before the inclemency of the feafons commenced, the following confequences would necefarily arife. Firft, Thofe animals whofe conftitutions were not formed to withftand the feverities of the frigid zone, would certainly perifh. Secondly, Thofe which furvived would become natives of the climates favourable to their exiftence. Such were the effects produced by the great change in the temperature of air.

A fimilar inftance happened in the year 1739, occafioned by that long and fevere froft. The weftern coaft of England being plentifully ftored with fcollop fhell-fifh ; it was obferved, that the fpecies almoft totally perifhed by the inclemency of that long feafon. ---This I had from good authority.

To fuch like caufes we may afcribe the deftruction of various fpecies of animals and vegetables, in diffe-

R   rent

rent regions of the earth, fubfequent to the grand convulfion.

Thefe circumftances being duly confidered, I prefume, it will appear, that the *exuviæ* of marine animals found remote from their native climates, are fo many inconteftible evidences of the alterations produced in the conftitution of the atmofphere at the time of the deluge ; and not as teftimonies of the deluge itfelf : for, in the firft inftance, it cannot be fuppofed that a bed of oyfters, &c. could have been removed two or three thoufand miles from their native climates, in the fpace of two or three months. And, fecondly, it is repugnant to common fenfe, and common experience, to fuppofe they could have been removed with fo much order, as to form diftinct beds of oyfters, cockles, &c. as living fifh do in the ocean.

Other inftances might be given to fhew the improbability of fuch effects being produced ; but we prefume, the above may fuffice to explode the idea of their having been brought from diftant regions by a flood , and alfo to convince us, that the alterations in the conftitution of the climates, and the deluge itfelf, were undoubtedly effects of the fame caufe, and produced at one and the fame time, as reprefented in chap. xii. and xiii.

3   As

As the fubject immediately under confideration feems to be a very interefting branch of natural hiftory. I hope it will merit a particular attention from my learned readers : conceiving it may throw fome light upon the learning and philofophy of the ancients, with refpect to the temperature and fertility of the firft ages, as reprefented by Hefiod, Ovid, and others.

Before we conclude this chapter, it may not be improper to recite fome inftances of animal remains being found remote from their native climates, as a corroborating teftimony of the preceding conclufions.

A CATALOGUE *of* EXTRANEOUS FOSSILS, *fhewing where they were dug up ; alfo their native Climates. Moftly felected from the curious Cabinet of Mr.* NEILSON, *in* King-ftreet, Red-Lion Square.

Their Names and Places where found.	Native Climates.
CHAMBERED NAUTILUS. Sheppy Ifland ; Richmond in Surrey; Shelborne in Dorfetfhire - - - -	*Chinefe Ocean and other Parts of that great Sea*
TEETH OF SHARKS. Sheppy Ifland, Oxfordfhire, Middlefex, Surrey, Northamptonfhire - - - -	*Eaft and Weft Indies.*

SEA

Their Names and Places where found.   Native Climates.

SEA TORTOISE, several kinds ; the *Hawksbill, Loggerhead,* and *Green* Species. Sheppy Island - - - } *West Indies.*

MANGROVE TREE OYSTERS. Sheppy Island - - - - .. } *West Indies.*

COXCOMB TREE OYSTERS. Oxford-shire, Gloucestershire, Dorsetshire, and Hanover - - - - - } *Coast of Guinea.*

VERTEBRÆ, *and* PALATES *of the* ORBES. Sheppy Island, and many other parts of England - - } *East and West Indies.*

CROCODILE. *Germany,* Derbyshire, Nottinghamshire, Oxfordshire, and Yorkshire, - - - }

ALLIGATOR's TEETH. Oxfordshire, Sheppy Island - - } *East and West Indies.*

The BANDED BUCCINUM. Oxford-shire, and the Alps - } *West Indies.*

The DIPPING SNAIL, and STAR FISH. Sheppy Island - - - } *West Indies.*

TAIL BUCCINUM. Sheppy Island, Hordel Cliff, Hampshire - } *East Indies.*

Now

Now fince it appears, that the *exuviæ* of marine animals are found remote from their native climates, and accompanied with a variety of circumftances, fhewing that they were actually generated in the climates where they are found ; it appears highly probable that thofe climates were originally fuitable to the nature of their exiftence.*

The antediluvian world was therefore more univerfally adapted to animal life, than the poftdiluvian ftate of Nature.

Confidering the great diverfity of feafons before and after the flood, leads me to inquire into their different effects on the period of human life, in the enfuing chapter.

---

* The preceding catalogue of animal *exuviæ* is principally felected from the marine creation, as they are more immediately in a ftate of freedom to inhabit thofe regions moft agreeable to them, than the terreftrial fpecies.

C H A P.

CHAP. XV.

On the Longevity of the Human Species before and after the Flood.

ACCORDING to the preceding chapters xii. xiii. and xiv. the following phenomena plainly appear.

Firſt, That mountains and continents emerged from beneath the deep at the time of the deluge.

Secondly, That the burning heats in the torrid zone, and the intenſe cold in the frigid zone, are not wholly owing to their reſpective ſituations, but rather to thoſe immenſe tracts of land, the *continents*.

Thirdly, That the temperature of the air and ſeaſons, in the antediluvian world, were leſs ſubject to extremes of heat and cold, and more univerſally adapted to *animal* and *vegetable life*, than the preſent conſtitution of Nature.

Theſe conſiderations lead me to inquire into their different effects on the period of human life.

1. It is a truth commonly known, that temperate climates are more friendly to animal and vegetable life,

than

than thofe which are fubject to great and fudden changes, fiom one extreme of heat and cold to another.

Hence, 1 prefume, invalids are fent to recruit their conftitutions in a more temperate air, and feldom fail of being benefited by the change of climate.   May we not therefore conclude, that if a temperate air has a tendency to reftore a weakly conftitution, that it muft certainly contribute to prolong the life of an healthy one.

To this purpofe Dr. Burnet obferves, in his Sacred Theory, vol. i. p. 275, 276.   " I know no place," fays he, " wheie the people live longer than in the *lit-* " *tle ifland* of *Bermudas.*   According to the pioportion " tion of time they hold out there, aftei they aiiive " fiom other parts of the woild, one may ieafonably " fuppofe that the natives would live two hundred " years , and yet nothing appeais in that ifland that " fhould give long life above other places, but the " extiaordinaiy fteadinefs of the weathei, and tempe- " iatuie of the air thioughout the whole yeai, fo that " theie is fcaice any difference of feafons."

Loid Bacon likewife remarks, that " iflanders aie, " for the moft pait, longer lived than thofe that live " on continents : for they live not fo long in Ruffia

" as

" as in the Orcades ; nor fo long in Africa, though in
" the fame parallel of latitude, as in the Canaries and
" Terceras ; and the Japonians are longer lived than
" the Chinefe, though the Chinefe are made for long
" life.   And this is no wonder," fays his Lordfhip,
" feeing the *air* of the *fea* doth *heat* and *cherifh* in
" *cooler regions*, and *cool* in *hotter*.

" The countries which have been obferved to pro-
" duce *long livers* are thefe, Arcadia, Ætolia, India
" on this fide the Ganges, Brafil, Taprobane, Britain,
" Ireland, with the iflands of the Orcades and He-
" brides."   See Hiftory on Life and Death, p. 21.

Italy is generally confidered as a more temperate climate than that of England, and productive of greater
longevity , though we have many long-lived people in
Britain.   The above noble author has recited many
inftances of great longevity in Italy, as follows :

" The year of our Lord feventy-fix, the reign of
" Vefpafian, is memorable ; for in that year there
" was a taxing.   Now taxing is the moft authentic
" method of knowing the age of men.   In that part
" of Italy, lying betwixt the Apennine mountains and
" the river Po, there was found an hundred and twen-
" ty-four perfons that either equalled, or exceeded, an
" hundred years of age : namely,

" Fifty

I

" Fifty-four - - - 100 years each.
Fifty-seven - - - 110
Two - - - - - 125
Four - - - - - 130
Four - - - - - 135 or 137
Three - - - - - 140

" Besides the above, Parma contained five ; whereof,

Three were - - - - 120 years each.
Two - - - - 130

One, in Bruxells - - 125
One, in Placentia - - 131
One in Faventia - - 132

" A town near Placentia, ten ; whereof

Six were - - - - 110 years each.
Four - - - - - 120

One in Rimino - - 150, whose name was
Marcus Aponius."

His Lordship has also enumerated many other people of much greater longevity than the above, but does not consider the records of them as equally authenticated with the former : therefore let the above suf-

S

fice,

fice, to fhew that temperate climates are productive of *long life.*

England and Ireland contain many inftances of great longevity ; but probably cannot boaft of fo many old people exifting in any one æra, as we find there have been in Italy, though by the following table it appears that they contain more than could well be imagined.

A TABLE OF LONGEVITY.

Names of the People	Age.	Places of Abode	Living or dead.
Thomas Paire — — —	152	Shropfhire	Nov 16, 1635.
Henry Jenkins — — —	169	Yorkfhire	Dec 8, 1670.
Robert Montgomery — —	126	ditto —	Living in the year 1670.
Anonymous — — —	140	ditto —	} Both living 1664.†
His Son — — — —	100	ditto —	
The Countefs of Defmond	140	Ireland —	
Mr. Eclefton — — —	143	ditto —	1691.
J. Sagar — — —	112	Lancafhire	1668 ‡
—— Lawrence —	140	Scotland —	Living '
Simon Sack — —	141	Frionia —	May 30, 1764
Col Thomas Winfloe —	146	Ireland —	Auguft 22, 1766.
Francis Confift — — —	150	Yorkfhire	January 1768.
Chriftian Jacob Drakenberg	146	Norway —	June 24, 1770.[2]
Margaret Forfter — —	136	Cumberland	} Living, 1771.
Her daughter — —	104	ditto —	
Francis Bons — — —	121	France —	Feb. 6, 1769.
John Brookey — — —	134	Devonfhire	Living, 1777.[3]
James Bowels — — —	152	Kilinworth*	Auguft 15, 1656.
John Tice — — —	125	Worcefterfh	March 1774.[4]
John Mount — — —	136	Scotland —	February 27, 1776.[5]
A goldfmith — — —	140	France —	June 1776[6]
Mary Yates — — —	128	Shropfhire	—— 1776.[7]

† And attended to give Evidence at York Affizes.
 * In Warwickfhire.
 ‡ See Philof. Tranf vol. iii. p. 306, 307, 308, 309 Lowthorp's Abr
 ' Derham's Phyfico-Theol. p 173.

[2] Annual Regifter, p 18 ;.
[3] Daily Advertifer, Nov. 18, 1777.
[4] Ibid, March 1774
[5] Morning Poft, Feb 29, 1776.
[6] Daily Advertifer, June 24, 1776.
[7] Ibid, Auguft 22, 1776.

The

The accounts borrowed from the public papers were collected by a gentleman whofe veracity may be relied on, though he unfortunately omitted fome of the authorities.

We may add to the preceding obfervations, that the natives of America are fhorter lived than thofe of England ; and that a Britifh conftitution will laft longer in America than a native one. This information may be relied on as a matter of fact.

Now fince it appears that temperate climates are conducive to long life in the poftdiluvian world, is it not reafonable to fuppofe, from the unalterable laws of Nature, that the fame caufe produced the fame effect before the flood ? and if fo, the prefumption is great that the antediluvians lived to a much greater age than the poftdiluvians ? for as a more univerfal temperature prevailed over the different regions of the earth in the former ftate of Nature, than does in the latter, may we not thence conclude, that the longevity of the antediluvians muft greatly exceed that of the poftdiluvian race of men ?

And more efpecially when we again confider, that our firft parents were brought into the world with conftitutions perfectly free from all thofe taints and impurities which the latter inherit from the intemperate

S 2

modes

modes of life in preceding ages, and at the same time provided with food, the most suitable to the nature of their existence.

From these considerations it appears highly probable, that if so many of the postdiluvians survive the age of an hundred and thirty or an hundred and forty, under the disadvantages of constitution, climate, &c. the antediluvians must certainly have survived the age of several hundred, according to the Scripture account.

Other circumstances apparently concurred in favour of the antediluvian longevity : namely that universal temperature which prevailed over the earth in the first ages, and the succulent state of its surface, are circumstances which would apparently produce great luxuriancy in the vegetable kingdom, and suffice the calls of human nature without art and labour ; therefore no anxious cares or jealousies invaded their repose ; property and dominion being then unknown, men past away their time in perfect security ; therefore, as harmony thus universally prevailed both in the heavens and the earth, it would certainly favour the longevity of our first parents, or stretch out their lives greatly beyond the reach of human conception.

But, alas ! the production of mountains and continents at the time of the deluge, put a final period to
that

that univerfal harmony which prevailed over the ante-diluvian world.   The burning heats of the torrid zone, and feverities of the frigid zone, were then brought forth : thus were men under the neceffity of protect-ing themfelves from the inclemency of the feafons, by building huts, or inhabiting caverns under ground. Neceffity, therefore, may be confidered as the parent of property, dominion, &c.   Such were apparently the confequences arifing from the great change in the con-ftitution of the atmofphere, at the time of that dreadful convulfion of Nature.

From that æra, the period of human life gradually contracted to its prefent ftandard , and, for the fame reafon that a conftitution removed from a temperate to an intemperate climate, will laft longer in the latter than a native conftitution ; for the fame reafon, an antedi-luvian conftitution would wear longer in the poftdi-luvian world, than thofe born after the flood.

Having thus confidered the longevity of the antedi-luvians, and the contraction of human life after the flood ; let us take a view of the ancient records, and obferve the analogy between the former and the latter.

Before

Before the Flood.	Years	After the Flood	Years	
Adam — — —	930	Noah after the flood —	350	=950
Seth — — —	912	Shem after the flood —	502	=600
Enos — — —	905	Arphaxad — —	438	
Cainan — — —	910	Salah — — —	403	
Mahalalul — —	895	Eber — — —	464	
Jared — — —	962	Peleg — — —	239	
Metheufelah — —	969	Reu — — —	239	
Lamech — — —	777	Serug — — —	230	
Noah before the flood	600	Nahor — — —	148	
Shem before the flood	98	Terah — — —	205	
		Abraham — —	175	
		Ifaac — — —	180	
		Jacob — — —	147	
		Jofeph* — — —	110	

Thus we find from the Mofaic account, that the *period* of *human life*, from Adam to Noah, continued nearly of the fame length ; and from the flood became gradually contracted to its prefent ftandard, in the fpace of 898 years, as in the inftance of Jofeph, all which perfectly coincides with the inferences deduced from the general laws of Nature, chap. xii, xiii, xiv.

Such are the periods of human life before the flood, according to Sacred writ : and though they cannot be truly afcertained from phyfical *data* ; yet it muft be owned, that the caufes affigned for the longevity of the

* 898 years after the flood.

ante-

antediluvians, have fome foundation in Nature ; and therefore, future difcoveries may poffibly give this rea-foning a lafting foundation. However that may be, the great analogy between revelation and reafon, may be confidered as corroborating the truth of each.

C H A P.

CHAP. XVI.

Concerning the Appearance of the Rainbow, after the Flood.

HAVING inquired into the ftate of the atmofphere in the antediluvian world, and its effects on the period of human life, let us extend our refearches a little further, and endeavour to afcertain the æra when the rainbow firft appeared.

That phenomenon is well known to arife from rays of light being refracted from fpherical drops of rain defcending towards the earth : therefore the appearance of the rainbow dependeth on there being *rain* or *no rain* before the *flood*.

Now according to the preceding chapters, the antediluvian atmofphere was more conftant and uniform in its temperature, and more homogeneous than that in the poftdiluvian world : for in the former there were no fiffures or volcanos to impregnate the air with noxious vapours ; nor continents to produce extremes of heat

and

3

and cold ; but harmony feems to have reigned univerfally over the new-formed globe.

Hence it appears, that the primitive ftate of the
earth was alfo more free from ftorms and tempefts than
the prefent ftate and condition of it, and confequently
more free from rain.

It is a general obfervation with mariners, that thofe
parts of the ocean the moft diftant from land are the
leaft fubject to ftorms and tempefts : nay, further,
that ftorms are a certain indication of its vicinity.

Don Antonia de Ulloa obferves, in his Voyage to
America, vol. i. p. 13, that " in the ocean, the winds
" are fo mild, that the motion of the fhip is hardly
" perceived, which renders the paffage extremely
" agreeable. The atmofphere of the ocean," fays he,
" anfwers to the calmnefs of the winds and fea ; fo
" that it is very feldom an obfervation cannot be ta-
" ken either from the fun's being obfcured, or the ha-
" zinefs of the horizon."

Varanius remarks, that " the winds are moft con-
" ftant in the Pacific Ocean, viz that part of it which
" lies between the tropicks , fo that the fhips which
" come from Aquapulco, a port in New Spain, in Ame-
" rica, to the Philipine Iflands, that is from eaft to weft,
" often fail three months, without ever changing or

T   " fhifting

" fhifting their fails ; having a conftant eaft or north
" eaft wind.   Nor did ever any fhip yet perifh in that
" vaft voyage of one thoufand fix hundred miles.   And
" therefore the failors think they may fleep there fe-
" curely : nor is there any heed of taking care of the
" fhip when that general wind carries them ftrait to
" their defired port, the Philipine Iflands.   And thus
" it is alfo in failing from the Cape of Good Hope, to
" Brafil in America, in the middle of which voyage lies
" the ifle of St. Helena." Varanius Geog. vol. i. p. 493.

" Dr. Halley, a perfon well fkilled in meteorology,
" as well as in all parts of phyfics, has, with extraordi-
" nary accuracy, profecuted the hiftory of the conftant
" periodical winds, which he deduces not only from the
" obfervations of feamen, but from his own experi-
" ence.   But he only takes notice of fuch winds
" as blow in the ocean ; there being fo much incon-
" ftancy and variablenefs in land winds, that from
" them a perfon can make out nothing clear or cer-
" tain."   See note to Varenius's Geog. vol. i. p. 496.

Now fince it appears that the atmofphere of the
ocean is uniform in its temperature, and conftantly
unruffled by ftorms and tempefts ; though the atmofphere of continents is continually fubject to violent
emotions,

emotions, and to great and fudden changes from one extreme of heat or cold to another ; may we not thence conclude, that thofe vaft tracts of land are the principal caufe of the former, as well as of the latter ? Therefore, as rain generally accompanies ftorms, it becomes highly probable, that they arife from one and the fame caufe, or, indeed, are infeparable.

Now as ftorms and tempefts only commenced with the production of mountains and continents, it feems to follow, that rain alfo commenced at the fame time.

Therefore, as an uniform temperature univerfally prevailed in the antediluvian atmofphere, it is highly probable it was not fubject to ftorms and tempefts, confequently not to *rain* ; and if there was no *rain*, there certainly could be no *rainbow*.

Thus the firft appearance of the rainbow feems to have commenced at the time of the deluge, with the production of mountains, continents, &c. Its appearance therefore, at that particular æra, is confiftent with the general order and progreffion of things.

It may, however be objected, that a want of rain for fo many hundred years, as from the creation to the deluge, would be greatly injurious, if not totally deftroy the vegetable kingdom : but we prefume fuch objec-

T 2

tions

tions will vanifh when the ftate and condition of the primitive iflands, is truly confidered.

1. The fcorching heats of fummer, and the feverities of winter, were not commenced.

2. The fuperficial contents of the iflands being fo much inferior to that of the continents, the furface of the fea, and the quantity of aqueous particles exhaled, were proportionably greater.

3. The atmofphere being thus more plentifully faturated with humidity, the latter defcended more copioufly in dews, during the abfence of the fun, and abundantly replenifhed the earth , rendered its furface foft and fucculent, and its vegetable productions luxuriant.

Such being apparently the ftate and condition of the antediluvian world, we cannot fuppofe that *rain* was in the leaft neceffary, either for the animal or the vegetable creation : and therefore, during that long period, it is highly improbable there fhould have been either *rain*, or a *rainbow :* for as the caufes productive of rain only commenced at the time of the deluge, may we not conclude, that the appearance of the rainbow could not precede that æra ?

Having now completed my inquiries into the original ftate and formation of the earth, and the changes it has undergone, I purpofe giving fome account of the

Derby-

Derbyſhire *ſtrata*, and their various productions of animal, vegetable and mineral fubſtances, as an illuſtration of the preceding chapters. And then ſhall conclude with a recapitulation of the work, as a means of throwing the fubject into one point of view.

APPEN-

APPENDIX.

Containing some general Observations on the Strata *in* Derbyshire, *with Sections of them, representing their* Arrangement, Affinities, *and the* Mutations *they have suffered, at different Periods of Time.*

THIS Appendix is intended, not only as an illustration of the preceding inquiries, but also as a specimen of Subterraneous Geography, a science of much importance to mankind, and not merely speculative, being applicable to the purposes of human life ; for by knowing the arrangement and affinities of the *strata*, we are enabled to investigate, with much certainty, whether coal or limestone are contained in the lower regions of the earth ; such is the general conformity of these things, so far as my observations have yet been extended. I would not be understood that the *strata* in every other part of the world are perfectly analogous to those in Derbyshire ; or that their productions are the same : but that there is as much regularity in the

2   arrange-

arrangement of the *ſtrata* in one country as there is in another : yet we have much reaſon to ſuppoſe that in ſome inſtances the *ſtrata* are univerſally analogous to each other, as will appear in the ſubſequent obſervations Having premiſed theſe matters, let us proceed to our obſervations on the Derbyſhire *ſtrata*.

Perhaps few parts of the world abound with a greater variety of natural phenomena than Derbyſhire ; on account of its mountains and mines, the ſingularity of its *ſtrata*, and their various productions of *animal*, *vegetable*, and *mineral* ſubſtances. The latter have occaſioned many ſhafts to be ſunk through the *ſtrata* at different depths, whereby the *number*, *thickneſs*, *quality*, and *poſition* of the *ſtrata*, have been obſerved with tolerable accuracy, and many other intereſting phenomena diſcovered.

Notwithſtanding the great antiquity of mining in Derbyſhire, it does not appear that any general obſervations on the *ſtrata*, &c. have yet been publiſhed, or ſo generally attended to as might be wiſhed, not only for the improvement of natural hiſtory, but that of mining in general. I am fully perſuaded in my own mind, that if the *ſtrata* in all mineral countries were faithfully repreſented by ſections, it would furniſh the miners with ſuperior ideas of their reſpective works, and enable them

to

to proceed in their works with more propriety. It would alfo be a peculiar fatisfaction to the proprietors of mines, to fee fections of the *ftrata*, with the nature or quality of each bed. To render thefe obfervations of more general utility to Subterraneous Geography, it would contribute much to regifter all *ftrata* cut through, and their productions, whether in digging for *copper*, *coals*, *lead*, *iron* or *water* ; for the moie general the obfervations, the more certain the inferences deduced from them.

In the fections annexed I have endeavoured to re-prefent the different qualities of the *ftrata* by hatched lines, &c. as colours are reprefented by the engiavers of coats of arms. I am very doubtful whether the mode I have chofen is the beft poffible for that purpofe, and fhould gladly receive any hints tending towards the im-piovement of fo valuable a branch of knowledge. It was my intention to have depofited fpecimens of each *ftratum*, with its productions, in the Britifh Mufeum, arranged in the fame order as they are in the earth, in-cumbent on each other ; being perfuaded that fuch a plan would convey a more perfect idea of Subterra-neous Geography, and of the various bodies contained in the earth, than words or lines can poffibly exprefs : and though I have not been able to complete this de-

U

fign

fign at prefent, I hope it may be done fome future day.

It is not my intention to enter into a minute defcription of the various ftones, minerals, petrefactions, &c. but rather to reprefent the general ftate and condition of the *ftrata*, and the changes they have undergone from various caufes. Neither do I affume to myfelf the fole honour of the following obfervations, having principally obtained them from feveral experienced miners; and particularly from Mr. George Tiffington, late of Winfter.

I have, indeed, very affiduoufly endeavoured to afcertain the truth of them by fubterraneous vifits, &c. and have alfo made fome difcoveries unnoticed by any other perfon before me: therefore, I am not confcious of any mifreprefentations, arifing either from neglect or a theoretical influence. I am not infenfible that much more remains to be done, and that in works of this nature, errors are unavoidable.

Plate I. reprefents a fection of the *ftrata* between Grange Mill and Darley Moor. The upper outline fhews the furface of the earth; the numbers 1, 2, 3, 4, &c. the refpective *ftrata*. Under the river Derwent is reprefented a fiffure filled up with rubble.

N° 1.

N° 1. MILLSTONE-GRET, 120 yards. A coarfe fandftone, compofed of granulated quartz and quartz pebbles. The former retain the fharpnefs of fragments newly broken, the latter are rounded as ftones on the fea fhore. This *ftratum* is not productive of minerals, nor figured ftones reprefenting any part of the animal or vegetable kingdoms.

The quartz pebbles contained in this *ftratum*, indicate a pie-exiftent ftate; for it is well known that quartz is a parafitical fubftance, formed in the fiffures of a quartzofe ftone, as fpar is formed in thofe of limeftone, and not in *ftrata*. This fhews that the pebbles were fift formed in fiffures; that the *ftrata* were broken, and their fragments rounded by attrition, as ftones on the fea beach, or in rivers.

The quartz pebbles abovementioned are white; the colour of the quartzofe ftones from whence they are produced is black, brown, &c. They are in common ufe for paving ftreets, and are frequently variegated with feams of white quartz running through them. They are the common gravel ftone of Nottinghamfhire, Staffordfhire, Derbyfhire, &c.

Quartzofe ftone is analogous to flint; it ftrikes fire with fteel, and refifts acids. It is lefs hard than flint, and breaks with a rough furface.

U 2

We

We are told that the minerals in Norway and Sweden are contained in the fiffures of a quartzoze ftone.

N° 2. SHALE or SHIVER, 120 yards. A black laminated clay, much indurated, contains neither animal nor vegetable impreffions, and is not confidered as a *ftratum* productive of minerals, as lead ore, fpar, &c. though an inftance or two has appeared to the contrary, in a mine called Shaw-Engine, near Eyam, attended with a curious circumftance. A vein of lead ore in N° 3, afcended into N° 2, fifteen or twenty fathoms; and the higher it afcended, the lefs and lefs it was mineralized, till it terminated in a white mucus-like fubftance. I had this information from people of veracity.

Quære. Was the ore generated from the mucus-like fubftance? or was that fubftance the product of ore decompofed by the acid contained in that *ftratum*?

The above *ftratum* contains ironftone in nodules, and fometimes ftiatified. The fprings iffuing from it aie of the chalybeate kind: for inftance, one near the bridge at Buxton, one at Quarndon, and another beyond Matlock Bridge, towards Chatfworth.

N° 3. LIMESTONE, 50 yards. Productive of lead ore, the oie of zinc, calamine, pyrites, fpar, fluoi, cauk, and cheit. This *ftratum* alfo contains figured ftones, reprefenting vaiious kinds of marine animals; as a gieat variety

variety of *anomiæ bivalves*, not known to exist in the British seas ; also *coralloids, entrochi* or screw-stones. I do not recollect ever seeing any univalves.

The impression of a crocodile was found in the above bed of stone, at Ashford, by Mr. Henry Watson of Bakewell.

The above *stratum* is composed of various *laminæ*, more or less separated by shale or shiver, a substance similar to N° 2 ; especially the upper, which are a good black, take a fine polish, and are thence called black marble. The lower *laminæ* are rather brown, as may be observed in the rocks composing Matlock High-Tor.

The ore of zinc is commonly called black-jack and mock-ore, from its similitude to lead ore. It is but lately discovered to contain zinc. When compounded with copper it makes brass, as calamine. Calamine, though similar in its mineral qualities, is apparently a simple brown earth ; it is commonly used in medicine by the name of *lapis calaminaris*.

N° 4. Toadstone, 16 yards. A blackish substance, very hard ; contains bladder-holes, like the *scoria* of metals, or Iceland *lava*, and has the same chymical property of resisting acids. Some of its bladder-holes are filled with spar, others only in part, and others again are quite empty. This *stratum* is not laminated, but

con-

confifts of one intire folid mafs, and breaks alike in all directions. It does not produce any minerals, or figured ftones reprefenting any part of the animal or vegetable creation, nor any adventitious bodies inveloped in it ; but is as much an uniform mafs as any vitrified fubftance whatever can be fuppofed to be : neither does it univerfally prevail, as the limeftone *ftrata*; nor is it, like them, equally thick ; but in fome inftances varies in thicknefs from fix feet to fix hundred, as will be fhewn hereafter. It is likewife attended with other circumftances which leave no room to doubt of its being as much a *lava* as that which flows from Hecla, Vefuvius, or Ætna.

The various circumftances relative to this apparent lava will be confidered in their due place, with fome attempt to inveftigate the caufe of its introduction between the limeftone *ftrata* ; and to fhew why it did not overflow the furface of the earth, according to the ufual operations of volcanos ?

It muft be obferved, that the above *ftratum* is known by the following names of *black-ftone* and *toad-ftone* at Matlock and Winfter ; at Moneyafh and Tidefwell, by that of *channel* ; and at Caftleton, by that of *catdirt*.

Nº 5. LIMESTONE, 25 fathoms. This *ftratum* is laminated like the former, Nº 3, and contains all the
fame

fame kinds of minerals and figured ftones. It is likewife productive of the Derbyfhire marble, fo much efteemed for its beauty and excellence in flabs and chimney-pieces. It abounds more plentifully with *entrochi*, or fcrew-ftone, than any other marine productions. The quarry from whence this marble is commonly raifed, is fituate on Moneyafh Moor, near the road, between that town and Bakewell ; its colour is grey.

N° 6. TOADSTONE, 23 fathoms. This *ftratum* is fimilar to N°4, in colour and chemical properties , but yet more folid, and freer from bladder holes, as may be obferved in Mofey-Meer mine, near Winfter.

N° 7. LIMESTONE, 30 fathoms. Laminated like the former N° 3 and 5, and like them contains minerals, and figured ftones ; but fewer of the latter. Its colour is much whiter than N° 5.

N° 8. TOADSTONE, 11 fathoms. This *ftratum* is fimilar to N° 6, but yet more folid, as may be obferved in Hubberdale mine, near Moneyafh.

N° 9. LIMESTONE, not yet cut through. Productive of minerals and figured ftones, like the former, N° 3, 5, and 7, but very few of the latter.

N. B. No VEGETABLE FORMS HAVE YET BEEN DISCOVERED IN ANY OF THE LIMESTONE STRATA.

Such

Such are the *strata*, their *productions*, *qualities*, and *characters* by which they are reprefented plate I. and it is neceffary to obferve further, that the fame characters are applied to exprefs the fame qualities, in all the other fections.

To the above we may add fix other *strata*, which are too minute to be expreffed on the fame fcale : thefe are ufually called *clays*, or *way-boards* ; in general they are not more than four, five, or fix feet thick, and in fome inftances not more than one foot. Their colour is a lightifh blue, with a fmall tint of green ; they all contain pyrites and fpar in fmall nodules ; and it has been obferved by Mr. George Tiffington, that all the fprings flowing from them are warm, like thofe of Buxton and Matlock-Bath. Thefe clays are calcarious, and may therefore be claffed with marles. They are arranged in the following order :

The firft *stratum* of clay feparates N° 3 and 4 ; the fecond, N° 4 and 5 ; the third, N° 5 and 6 ; the fourth, N° 6 and 7 ; the fifth, N° 7 and 8 ; the fixth, N° 8 and 9. By thefe clays the thicknefs of the other *strata* is afcertained, which otherwife would be difficult, as the limeftone beds confift of various *laminæ*.

Having defcribed the *strata*, and their various productions contained in plate I. let us take a general

view

view of them. 1ft. It is to be obferved that this fection is only intended to reprefent the arrangement of the *ftrata*, and not all the particular circumftances accompanying them, with refpect to their feveral fractures, diflocations, &c.

To proceed. The lower *ftrata* appear on the furface on Bonfal Moor, and the upper in the valley : for inftance, N° 2, on the banks of the river Derwent ; N° 3, in Trogues-pafture ; N° 4, 5, 6, 7, and 8, on Bonfal Moor, although the elevation of that mountain cannot be lefs than eight hundred or a thoufand feet above the level of the river Derwent.

When the lower *ftrata* thus appear at the furface, they are faid to baffet.

What has been obferved of the lower *ftrata* baffeting on Bonfal Moor, is likewife true in many other parts of Derbyfhire. For inftance :

Stratum N° 2, appears in the vallies of Bakewell, Afhford, and Caftleton , and likewife on Mam-Tor, although that mountain is nearly a thoufand feet above the level of Caftleton valley. N° 4 forms the fummit of a mountain adjacent to the caftle, and is there called *cat-d.rt*.

N° 5 forms the furface of Moneyafh Moor, at the marble quarry ; and likewife at Hubberdale-

mine,.

mine, although that mountain, by computation, is feven or eight hundred feet above the level of Bakewell or Afhford.

Let us now take a view of plate II. which reprefents a fection of the *ftrata* at Matlock High-Tor. N° 1, 2, 3, 4, 5, &c. on each fide the river, fhew the corefponding *ftrata*; whence it appears that they have been *burft*, *diflocated*, and *thrown* into *confufion*, by fome violent convulfion of Nature.

The *ftrata* which compofe the top of Maffon Mountain, are elevated about one hundred fathoms above the fummit of Matlock High-Tor, N° 3; and the fame beds are depreffed about fifty fathoms below the foot of it, at the river, as fhewn in the plate. A, reprefents a great *fiffure* or *chafm*, filled up with the *fragments* of the *upper* and *adjacent ftrata*.

Such is the general ftate of the mountainous part of Derbyfhire, which perfectly coincides with the refult of chap. xii. p. 88, 89: and therefore, ferves to fhew the effects produced by fubterraneous convulfions, and that mountains are not primary productions of Nature, but of a very diftant period of time from the creation of the world.

Whence it appears, that all fuch vallies were originally great gulfs or fiffures thus filled up. Therefore,

fore, as the *strata*, N° 1 and 2, have totally disap-
peared on the weft fide of the river, together with a
part of N° 3, the prefumption is great that they have
been thus fwallowed up into that enormous cleft ,
and if in this inftance, the fame thing may have
happened in many others ; if not univerfally, in all
mountainous countries, wherein the upper *strata*
have difappeared. For in Derbyfhire, wherever
miners have occafion to dig in vallies, they find them
thus filled up with fragments of the fuperior beds.

It may appear ftrange to our imagination, that
fuch immenfe maffes of earth fhould have been thus
totally abforbed into the bowels of the earth ; but
when we confider the probability of thefe gulfs being many miles or many hundreds of miles deep,
fee chap. xii. it will no longer remain a matter of
wonder what is become of the fuperincumbent *stra-*
ta, fo often miffing amongft the mountains , but
rather that thofe horrid chafms fhould have been fo
nearly filled up.

R, reprefents a mine called High - Tor-Rake.
B, B, B, the correfponding fiffures, feparated by beds
of toadftone.

But when I fpeak of incumbent beds, I do not
confine myfelf to thofe of millftone grit, and fhale,

but

but include thofe of argillaceous ftone, clay and coal : for according to plates III IV. VI. wherever *ftratum* N° 1, dips, or difappears, as there reprefented, thofe of argillaceous ftone, clay, and coal, become the incumbent beds : therefore, fince this obfeivation holds univerfally true in Derbyfhire, it feems highly probable, that the *ftrata* of *clay*, *coal*, &c. have been originally incumbent on *grit*, and were fwallowed up by that dreadful convulfion which burft the *ftrata* and threw them into all this diforder. However that might have been, fuch is the ftate of them ; therefore I leave the reader to draw his own conclufions.

Let us now return to plate I. A, A, A, and G, G, G, G, reprefent the correfponding fiffures in the limeftone *ftrata*, interfected by beds of folid toadftone. All the fiffures thus correfpond in the limeftone *ftratu* in Derbyfhire; not a fingle inftance knowingly, has happened to the contraiy ; but it does not follow that they aie all thus inteifected ; for we have many inftances wheie the *ftrata* N° 4, and 6, do not exift, as will be fhewn heieafter : neither are they equally thick, as repiefented in the fection, although the upper and lower fuifaces of the othei *ftrata*, are nearly parallel, but more of this in its due place.

It

It is a general obfervation, and invariably true, that minerals are only contained in the *fiſſures* of *limeſtone ſtrata*, and between their *laminæ*, and *not in* the *ſolid ſubſtance* of the *ſtone*.

When they are difcovered in the fiſſures, the mines are called rake-works : when between the *laminæ*, pipe-works.

The following mines are inſtances of the feveral limeſtone *ſtrata* producing lead-ore.

Yate-ſtoop in *ſtratum* - - - -	N° 3.
Portaway and Placket in - - -	N° 5.
Moſey-meer in - - - - - -	N° 7.
Gorſey-dale in - - - - - -	N° 9.

All the *ſtrata*, except toadſtone, may be confidered as equally thick, when covered by an incumbent bed ; but when expoſed to the operations of the air, they are greatly diminiſhed in thickneſs, decompoſed as it were, and changed to a vegetable mould, whether *grit*, *limeſtone*, or *toadſtone*.

And it is obfervable, that the effects of the weather extend many feet below the furface of the earth. Immediately under the foil, the fragments of the ſtone are fmall, and gradually increafe in bulk to the depth of fifteen or twenty feet, where the *ſtratum* generally becomes folid, and fit for the mafon.

We

We have now to obferve of the *ftrata* in general, that wherever N° 1 appears on the furface, N° 2 lies certainly underneath it. And where N° 2 forms the furface, N° 3 is the fucceeding *ftratum*, and this holds true with all the other *ftrata*, where any ob-fervations have been made, the toadftone excepted : and therefore fince grit and fhale are now only to be found in broken detached parts, difperfed over the mountainous parts of Derbyfhire : it appears highly probable, that they have originally prevailed over that part of the country, according to our obferva-tions on the argillaceous ftones, p. 155, 156.

Let us now take fome notice of the toad-ftone, fince it appears to have been formed by a dif-ferent caufe.

We have already obferved, that toadftone inter-fects the mineral veins, and totally cuts off all communication between the upper and the lower fiffures.

Hence it is that when a mineral vein in N° 3, is cut down to N° 4, all mineral appearances totally vanifh.

But experience, the great mafter in phyfical refearches, has taught the miner to dig through the toadftone to the limeftone N° 5, where he never fails finding the correfponding vein.

The

The above facts are univerfally true ; and therefoie merit a particular attention, as they will be called forth hereafter, to prove the origin of toadftone

Another circumftance accompanying toad-ftone, is, the clofenefs of its texture , a property of great utility in the piactice of mining : for in-ftance, fuppofe the fprings in a mine at I, plate I. near Wenfley, were either too powerful, to be iaifed by an engine, or the expence of raifing them too great, the work then ftands, and a fhaft is funk at an upper level at O, down to N° 5 at *a*, and a gate or gallery diiven under N° 4 to the correfponding fiffure at G. This is a common practice amongft the miners in Derbyfhire, and never fails pioducing a diy work in *ftratum* N° 5 , for the clofe textuie of the toad-ftone will not filtrate water fufficient to incommode the woik-men, although it may be ten or fifteen fa-thoms deep in N° 3, as iepiefented by the hoiizontal line L, L. This circumftance likewife fhews that the toadftone is free from fiffuies.

Anothei ciicumftance accompanying toadftone, is, that it fiequently fills up fiffuies of the limeftone *ftrata* lying immediately under it, (See S. H. plate I.) more or lefs, as they are more or lefs wide. When

2

fiffuies

fiſſures are thus filled up, the miners call it *troughing*. Two ſuch inſtances have been diſcovered on Bonſal Moor; one of them in the mine called *Slack*; the other in that called *Salters-way*. In the former there are two fiſſures which interſect each other, called a croſs-rake. One of them contains toadſtone, the other minerals. See plate **IX.** fig. 2. A, B, the mineral vein, totally ſeparated by the toadſtone F, F.

It is neceſſary further to obſerve, that a ſhaft was ſunk at this mine forty or fifty fathoms deep in toadſtone, and no bottom yet found. Another ſhaft was ſunk about ſixty yards from the former, ſuppoſe towards the eaſt, and the ſame toadſtone was found about twenty fathoms thick. Another ſhaft was alſo ſunk about the ſame diſtance towards the weſt, and the toadſtone was found near twenty fathoms thick.* Theſe circumſtances ſeem to ſhew, that the firſt ſhaft was ſunk in a fiſſure.

Similar inſtances are not uncommon, therefore the above may be conſidered as characteriſtic of the mineral part of Derbyſhire.

In the mine called Salters-way, a fiſſure has been diſcovered in part filled up with toadſtone, and in

* I was favoured with the above obſervations from Thomas Pounder, of Bonſal, an intelligent miner.

part with the fragments of limeftone, minerals, &c. See the fection, plate **IX.** fig. 3. F, F, F, reprefents the toadftone.

On Tidefwell Moor, the toadftone, or channel, as there called, has been dug one hundred fathoms deep, and no bottom found; though in feven other mines adjacent, the fame *ftratum* has been dug through, and its thicknefs afcertained at each place, as under.

Names of the Mines.	*Fathoms.*
A. Black Hillock - - -	100 not cut through.
B. Heath Bufh - - - -	16 cut through.
C. St. Andrew's - - - -	2 ditto.
D. St. James's - - - -	12 ditto.
E. Conftant - - - - -	7 ditto.
F. Calveftone - - - - -	7 ditto.
G. Dunkirk - - - - -	19 ditto.
H. Chap-maiden - - - -	17 ditto.

Plate **VII.** fhews the fituation of each fhaft where the obfervations were made, by Mr. William Haigh of Tidefwell.

The above may ferve to fhew that toadftone is fo extremely variable in its thicknefs, as not to admit of being truly reprefented by a fection Let us now
Y enume-

enumerate a few inftances where this ftone has not yet been found. viz.

In the mines at *Eyam, Foolow,* and *Afhover,* although thofe mines are funk near fifty fathoms in the limeftone ; and the *ftratum* N° 5, forms the furface of the earth at Foolow.

The *ftrata* N° 4 and 6, are not univerfal ; they have no exiftence in Hubeidale Mine, near Moneyafh ; Hangworm Mine on Bonfal Mooi ; nor at High-Rake Mine near Tidefwell, &c.

Hence it evidently appears, that toadftone is attended with many circumftances very different from the other *ftrata.* 1. It is peifectly fimilar to Iceland lava in its appearance and chymical quality. 2 It is extremely variable in its thicknefs. 3. It is not univerfal. 4. It has no correfponding fiffures to thofe in limeftone. 5. It frequently fills up the fiffures in the *ftratum* underneath it, more or lefs, as they are moie or lefs wide.

All thefe circumftances plainly evince, that toadftone was formed by a very different law from the otheis, and greatly pofterior to them ; for the beds of limeftone muft have been formed befoie they weie broken, and broken before their fiffures could have been filled up : therefore we may, with much reafon, conclude,

clude, that *toadstone, channel*, and *cat dirt*, is actual lava, and flowed from a volcano whose funnel, or shaft, did not approach the open air, but disgorged its fiery contents between the *strata* in all directions. Another remarkable phenomenon accompanying the Derbyshire lava is that the *stratum* of clay lying under N° 6, is apparently burnt, as much as an earthen pot or brick; insomuch that when compared to the burnt clay on Heynor Common, they are not to be distinguished asunder. The Heynor clay was burnt by a *stratum* of coal being on fire underneath it, and is the best material in that neighbourhood for the repair of public roads. Their stone though hard being all of it argillaceous, soon returns to its primitive clay by the pressure of coal carriages.

I have heard of many similar instances of the clay under N° 6 being in a calcined state, but I have only seen specimens of it from Mossey-meer Mine near Winster. The *stratum* of clay is about four feet thick, and thus burnt about one foot deep.

Having enumerated the various circumstances relative to the lava, there can be little doubt of its being actually a volcanic production. However probable that may appear, the intelligent reader may possibly ask by what process lava was introduced between such immense beds of stone?

Y 2 The

The queftion, I confefs, is more eafily ftated than anfwered, yet feems to require a folution to eftablifh the identity of its being lava.

We will, therefore attempt the inveftigation, difficult as it may appear : for fhould we fail in the attempt, future difcoveries may poffibly afford a more fatisfactory folution.

Previous to the inquiry, it is neceffary to obferve, that the introduction of lava between the limeftone *ftrata* was anterior to the fracture reprefented plate II. This is evident from the correfponding *ftrata* on each fide the river, and alfo from the fragments of the toadftone contained in the fiffure. Thefe circumftances likewife fhew that the pofition of the *ftrata* was altered by the convulfion which occafioned the fracture, whence we may infer they had originally an uniform arrangement, concentric to the center of the earth. And if in this inftance, may we not conclude, by analogy, that fince all the mountainous part of Derbyfhire is in a fimilar ftate of confufion ; that they have been difordered from a fimilar caufe ; and confequently all its *ftrata* muft have had originally an unifoim arrangement at the time lava was introduced between them.

This being granted, it will then follow, that the *ftrata* of grit and fhale, which are now only found in

broken

broken detached maffes, varioufly difperfed over the north part of Derbyfhire, univerfally prevailed, or were fuperincumbent on limeftone. And by parity of rea-fon, it will hold equally true, that the *ftrata* of argilla-ceous ftone, clay, and coal, reprefented plate III. IV. VI. weie alfo univerfally incumbent on grit. Such I conceive to have been the original ftate and con-dition of the *ftrata* prior to the convulfion which threw them into their prefent ftate of diforder.

Having premifed thefe matters, let us confider by what apparent caufe *lava* could have been introduced between the limeftone *ftrata*, at a time when they were compreffed by fuch an immenfe incumbent weight of fhale, grit, argillaceous ftone, clay, and coal; and likewife fhew why the *lava* did not burft open a paffage and overflow the furface of the earth.

Firft, According to chapter XII. fubteiraneous fire prevailed univerfally eithei in the fame *ftratum* or in the central part of the eaith, as reprefented plate IX. fig. 1.

Secondly, The expanfive force of this fiie *elevated*, and *burft* the incumbent *ftrata*, piior to the convulfion which threw them into their prefent ftate of confu-fion.

Fiffures,

Fiſſures being thus opened over the melted matter, the violent preſſure of the incumbent weight might cauſe it to aſcend till it met with an obſtruction ſuperior to the impelling force.

Let us now ſuppoſe, for the preſent, that the lava was thus circumſtanced : it would conſequently have a lateral preſſure proportionable to the impelling force ; and therefore might probably penetrate between the *ſtrata*, and force its way, till it loſt its fluidity by the coldneſs of the adjacent beds. Being thus extended to ſome diſtance, and paſſing over other fiſſures, it might fill them up more or leſs, as they happened to be more or leſs wide, and the lava more or leſs fluid.

Hence, I preſume, the fiſſures in the Salterway mine being only in part filled up with lava, was owing to the above cauſe. See plate IX. fig. 3, F F F the lava.

Now ſince it appears that the ſhaft in Black Hillock mine, was ſunk one hundred fathoms in lava, there is ſome probability that it flowed from the bowels of the earth, up that fiſſure, and ſpread itſelf laterally in all directions ; and this conjecture is ſtrengthened by the various thickneſſes of the ſame maſs of matter at the different mines, laid down in the plan plate VII.

We have now to conſider why the lava did not overflow the ſurface of the earth ?

It

It has already been obferved, that lava was introduced between the *ftrata* during their uniform arrangement, and whilft the beds of argillaceous ftone, clay, coal, grit, and fhale were univerfally incumbent on lime-ftone.

Now it feems highly probable that fhale, at fo remote a period, was a foft, ductile fubftance, more fubject to extenfion by an internal expanfive force, than to crack or break, like the limeftone, which was perfectly concreted : therefore fince that *ftratum* is one hundred and twenty yards thick, and was covered by a *ftratum* of grit of the fame thicknefs, and that grit by all the beds of argillaceous ftone, &c. amounting to feveral hundred yards more : it feems highly probable, that the united refiftance of fo much incumbent weight, together with the quantity and quality of the fhale, might totally obftruct the lava in its paffage towards the furface, and caufe it to fpread laterally between the limeftone *ftrata*.

Such are the conjectures which at prefent occur to me why the melted matter did not approach the furface of the earth, according to the ufual mode of volcanic operations.

Having now compleated my obfervations on the Derbyfhire lava, and on the general ftate and condi-

tion

tion of the *ſtrata* productive of lead-ore, &c. I pro-
poſe to enlarge my obſervation on the argillaceous
ſtrata productive of coal.

Plate III. repreſents a ſection of the *ſtrata*, eaſt and
weſt of the river Derwent, from Belper-Ward towards
Blackbrook.   In this ſection, N° 1 dips or diſappears
at the river, and thoſe of argillaceous ſtone, clay, and
coal become the ſuperior beds, and are characterized
accordingly.   For inſtance, *a a a a a a* repreſent the
argillaceous ſtone ; *b b b b b* clay, bind, or clunch,
ſynonymous terms ; *c c c* coal.   The upper *ſtratum*
of argillaceous ſtone is excellent for the uſe of cutlers'
grinding ſtones, and carpenters' whetſtones.   It is of
a browniſh colour, and may be obſerved in all the
roads about Smalley, Heynor, Denby, Heage, Pent-
ridge, Alfreton, Carnfield, Cheſterfield, Sheffield, &c.
It does not efferveſce with acids, and as it has already been obſerved, when applied to the repair of roads
ſoon returns to its primitive clay.

The lower *ſtrata* are much harder, will ſtrike fire
with ſteel, and are more durable and fit for the buſi-
neſs of the roads.   Theſe beds are more white, and are
commonly called crow-ſtone.

The

The beds of *clay, clunch,* or *bind,* are much indurated, and appear like ftone, but foon diffolve by the weather.

All the above *ftrata,* incumbent on coal, whether argillaceous ftone or clay, contain figured ftones reprefenting a great variety of vegetables, or the impreffions of them ; as reeds of various kinds, ftriated and jointed at different diftances. The *euphorbia* of the Eaft-Indies, the American ferns, corn, grafs, and many other fpecies of the vegetable kingdom. They are inclofed in the folid fubftance of the ftone, &c.

Thefe vegetable forms, and the *ftrata* containing them, are the certain indication of coal, not only in Derbyfhire, but in every part of this kingdom which I have vifited ; and I am informed, that the fame phenomenon holds equally true in every other part of the world yet explored.

Sir *Afhton Leaver's* incomparable *mufeum* of natural curiofities contains the moft perfect fpecimens and the greateft variety of foffil vegetables, if I may be allowed to call them fo, I ever faw.

Now fince it appears that all *ftrata* accompanying *coal* univerfally abound with vegetable forms, it feems to indicate that all coals were originally derived from the vegetables thus enveloped in the ftone or clay : and we

Z

may

may fay as much of the origin of iron ; for the fame *ſtrata* alfo produce iron-ftone.

It is a matter worthy notice, that the fuperior *ſtrata* contain iron-ftone, coals and vegetable impreffions ; and NO MARINE PRODUCTIONS WHATEVER. And that the inferior *ſtrata,* which are limeftone, contain the *exuviæ* of marine animals, &c. AND NO VEGETA-BLE FORMS WHATEVER.

Such is the arrangement of the *ſtrata* in Derbyfhire, fo far as my obfervations have been extended ; and not only in Derbyfhire, but in Staffordfhire, Shropfhire, &c.

We have now obtained fome general truths refpect-ing the conftruction of the earth, or the arrangement of its *ſtrata*, which may ferve to point out the proba-bility of coal or limeftone being contained in the lower regions of the earth.

1. That the coarfe millftone-grit, defcribed page 147, is never incumbent on coal, but always incum-bent on limeftone.

2. That argillaceous ftone is always incumbent on grit and coal.

Hence appears the neceffity of conftructing a mu-feum compofed of the different *ſtrata*, and their pro-ductions of animal, vegetable and mineral fubftances,

arranged

arranged in the fame order they are in the earth. This would convey a perfect idea of the bodies themfelves, and fhew us the order in which the refpective *ftrata* were fucceffively formed : for thofe containing marine productions only, muft ceitainly have been formed whilft the fea covered the earth, , and thofe containing vegetables, and no marine *exuviæ*, muft have been formed after the eaith became habitable. It is therefore apparently repugnant to the general courfe of Nature, that *terreftrial animals* and *vegetables* fhould be *blended together* with *marine productions*, in the *primary ftrata* of *limeftone*. The earth, indeed, has been ftrangely and fo frequently tumbled and toffed about, that without a particular attention to fuch circumftances, the general order may be apparently contradicted : of which the celebrated Mr. John Ray quotes a particular inftance. See his Three Difcourfes, 3d edit. p. 223.

" In the whole city of Modena, and round about
" for fome miles diftance, in whatever place they dig,
" when they come to the depth of about fixty-three
" feet, they pierce the ground with a *terebra* or au-
" ger, about five feet deeper, and then the water
" fpiings up with fo gieat force, that in a moment the
" well is filled up to the brim. This water is perpe-

Z 2 " tual,

" tual, doth not increase by rain, nor decrease by
" drought ; and, what is yet more remarkable, from
" the surface of the ground to the depth of fourteen
" feet, they meet with nothing but rubbish and ruins
" of an ancient city.   Being come to that depth,
" they found paved streets, artificers shops, floors of
" houses, and several pieces of inlaid-work.

" It is very hard to conceive how the ground of
" this city was raised thus ; we can attribute it to no-
" thing else, but that it hath been ruined, and after-
" wards rebuilt upon its ruins ; since it is not higher
" but rather lower still than all the adjacent country.

" After these ruins they find a very solid earth,
" which one would think had never been removed ;
" but a little lower they find it black and marshy, and
" full of briars.   Signor Rammazzini went down one
" of these wells, and at the depth of twenty-four
" feet he found a heap of wheat intire ; in another of
" twenty-six feet, he found filbert-trees, with their
" nuts.   They found likewise every six feet alternate-
" ly, a change of earth, sometimes white, with branch-
" es and leaves of trees of different sorts.

" At the depth of twenty-eight feet, or thereabouts,
" they find a chalk that cuts very easy.   It is mixed
" with shells of several sorts, and makes a bed of about
                                        " eleven

" eleven feet. After this they find a bed of marfhy
" earth, of about two feet, mixed with rufhes, leaves,
" and branches. After this bed comes another chalk
" bed of nearly the fame thicknefs with the former,
" which ends at the depth of forty-two feet.

" That is followed by another bed of marfhy earth
" like the former. After which comes a new chalk
" bed, but thinner, which hath alfo a marfhy bed un-
" derneath it. This ends at the place where the work-
" men bore with their auger. The bottom is fandy,
" mingled with a fmall gravel, in which they find fe-
" veral fhells, fuch as are on the fea-fhores.

" Thefe fucceffive beds of marfhy earth and chalk,
" are to be found in the fame order, in whatever parts
" of the earth you dig. The auger fometimes finds
" great trees, which give the workmen much trouble.
" They fee alfo, at fome times, at the bottom of thefe
" wells, great bones, coals, flints, and pieces of iron."

Thefe alternate beds of marfhy earth and chalk may
poffibly be confidered as a contradiction to what I conceive to be the general arrangement of the *ftrata*, viz.
that all *ftrata* productive of vegetable impreffions are
fuperior to thofe containing marine *exuviæ*. But the
only inference apparently to be deduced from the
ftrata at Modena is, that the fuperficial parts of the
earth, in fundry places, may have fuffered frequent alterations

terations from fea to land, and from land to fea ; and not that the *ftrata* in general were thus formed : therefore, fuch phenomena require a particular infpection before we can with propriety draw any conclufions from them refpecting the general order of the *ftrata*.

We have one inftance in Derbyfhire, fomewhat fimilar to the above ; namely, a *ftratum* of ironftone, plentifully abounding with the fhells of fifh : therefore, as ironftone is generated in the argillaceous beds, and thofe beds are fuperincumbent on grit, fhale, and limeftone, thefe *exuviæ* may alfo be confidered as a manifeft contradiction to the fuppofed general order ; but it is very eafy to obferve, that thefe fhells are not marine productions, but of frefh-water lakes, rivers, &c. being actually the remains of horfe mufcles.

The above *ftratum* of ironftone extends from Tupton Moor, near Wingerworth, the feat of Sir Henry Hunloke, Bart. to Stavely : it is about one foot thick, and lies about eight yards below the furface of the earth.

As a farther teftimony of the general conformity of the *ftrata*, plate V. reprefents a fection thereof at Lincoln Hill, near Colbrooke Dale, Shropfhire. N° 1, 1, 1, 1, *ftrata* of millftone-grit, fimilar to N° 1, in the Derbyfhire *ftrata*. N° 3, limeftone ; P P, *ftrata* of

quartz

quartz pebbles ; *a a a*, argillaceous ſtone ; *b b*, bind ; *c c*, coal.

The *ſtrata* about Colbrooke-Dale have been ſtrangely ſhattered to pieces, and thrown into great diſorder, as appears by the ſection. Both the argillaceous *ſtrata* and thoſe of limeſtone abound with a great variety of figured ſtones, the former repreſenting the vegetable kingdom, and the latter, the animal kind, of marine origin.

Plate VI. repreſents a ſection of the *ſtrata* from the new plantation in Chatſworth Old Park, to the river Derwent. The N° 1, 2, 3, &c. ſhew the correſponding *ſtrata* on each ſide a ſuppoſed great fiſſure , and ſhew that although there is a *ſtratum* of coal in the Old Park, there is none in the plantation ; owing to the diſarrangement of the *ſtrata*. Theſe are the circumſtances which render the practice of mining very uncertain, to thoſe who do not attend to the quality of the upper *ſtratum*.

Though the break here repreſented is not viſible, yet knowing the quality of the *ſtratum* N° 1, and that it is conſtantly inferior to that of coal, we may conclude with as much certainty that there is a break in the *ſtrata* as if it was viſible to the eye. Such is the invariable conformity in the courſe of Nature.

To

terations from fea to land, and from land to fea ; and not that the *ftrata* in general were thus formed : therefore, fuch phenomena require a particular infpection before we can with propriety draw any conclufions from them refpecting the general order of the *ftrata*.

We have one inftance in Derbyfhire, fomewhat fimilar to the above ; namely, a *ftratum* of ironftone, plentifully abounding with the fhells of fifh : therefore, as ironftone is geneiated in the argillaceous beds, and thofe beds are fuperincumbent on grit, fhale, and limeftone, thefe *exuviæ* may alfo be confidered as a manifeft contradiction to the fuppofed general order ; but it is very eafy to obferve, that thefe fhells are not marine productions, but of frefh-water lakes, iivers, &c. being actually the remains of horfe mufcles.

The above *ftratum* of ironftone extends from Tupton Moor, near Wingerworth, the feat of Sir Henry Hunloke, Bart. to Stavely : it is about one foot thick, and lies about eight yards below the furface of the earth.

As a farther teftimony of the general conformity of the *ftrata*, plate V. reprefents a fection thereof at Lincoln Hill, near Colbrooke Dale, Shropfhire. N° 1, 1, 1, 1, *ftrata* of millftone-grit, fimilar to N° 1, in the Derbyfhire *ftrata*. N° 3, limeftone ; P P, *ftrata* of

quartz

quartz pebbles ; *a a a*, argillaceous ftone ; *b b*, bind ; *c c*, coal.

The *ftrata* about Colbrooke-Dale have been ftrange-ly fhattered to pieces, and thrown into great diforder, as appears by the fection. Both the argillaceous *ftra-ta* and thofe of limeftone abound with a great variety of figured ftones, the former reprefenting the vegetable kingdom, and the latter, the animal kind, of marine origin.

Plate VI. reprefents a fection of the *ftrata* from the new plantation in Chatfworth Old Park, to the river Derwent. The N° 1, 2, 3, &c. fhew the correfpond-ing *ftrata* on each fide a fuppofed great fiffure ; and fhew that although there is a *ftratum* of coal in the Old Park, there is none in the plantation ; owing to the difarrangement of the *ftrata.* Thefe are the cir-cumftances which render the practice of mining very uncertain, to thofe who do not attend to the quality of the upper *ftratum.*

Though the break here reprefented is not vifible, yet knowing the quality of the *ftratum* N° 1, and that it is conftantly inferior to that of coal, we may conclude with as much certainty that there is a break in the *ftrata* as if it was vifible to the eye. Such is the in-variable conformity in the courfe of Nature.

To

To conclude, it is neceffary to obferve, that the *fec-tions* reprefenting the *ftrata* of *argillaceous ftone, clay,* and *coal,* are not laid down by the fame fcale with thofe of limeftone, &c. Twenty of the former being only equal in thicknefs to one of the latter, I have taken the liberty of reducing their numbers, and increafing their thicknefs, in order to diftinguifh their different qualities by hatched lines.

Therefore *nothing* more is intended to be underftood by them, but to fhew that they are univerfally incumbent on grit. Hence the following tables become neceffary to fhew their real dimenfions.

A TABLE

A TABLE *of the* STRATA *at* ALFRETON-COMMON.

Numb.		Feet.	Inches.
1	CLAY - - - - - - - - - -	7	0
2	RATCHELL, *fragments of ftone*	9	0
3	BIND, *indurated clay* - - - - -	13	4
4	STONE *argillaceous, or concreted clay* -	6	0
5	BIND - - - - - - - - -	8	8
6	BIND - - - - - - - - -	25	0
7	STONE, *a black colour* - - - - -	5	0
8	BIND - - - - - - - -	2	0
9	STONE - - - - - - - - -	2	0
10	BIND - - - - - - - -	5	0
11	BIND - - - - - - - - -	5	0
12	COAL - - - - - - - - -	1	6
13	BIND - - - - - - - -	1	6
14	STONE - - - - - - - -	23	0
15	STONE - - - - - - - -	14	0
16	BIND - - - - - - - -	7	0
17	SMUTT, *a black fubftance, refembling a ftratum of coal-duft* - - }	3	0
18	BIND - - - - - - - -	3	0
19	STONE - - - - - - - -	20	0
20	BIND - - - - - - - -	16	0
21	COAL - - - - - - - -	7	4
	A a	184	4

A TABLE *of the* STRATA *at* WEST-HALLAM.

Numb.		Feet.	Inches
1	CLAY	7	6
2	BIND	48	0
3	SMUTT	1	6
4	CLUNCH, *or indurated clay*	4	0
5	BIND	3	0
6	STONE	2	3
7	BIND	1	0
8	STONE	1	0
9	BIND	3	0
10	STONE	1	0
11	BIND	16	0
12	SHALE	2	0
13	BIND	12	0
14	SHALE	3	0
15	CLUNCH, *stone and sometimes cank*	54	0
16	SOFT COAL	4	0
17	CLAY	0	6
18	SOFT COAL	4	6
19	CLUNCH *and* BIND	21	0
20	COAL	1	0
21	BIND	1	0
22	*Strong, broad* BIND	25	0
23	COAL	6	0
		222	3

Altho' the preceding obfervations have a tendency to prove that coal is not to be found under a *ftratum* of limeftone, yet we have an inftance to the contrary at Etruria and Little Fenton, near Newcaftle in Staffordfhire, as follows :

Firft *ftratum*, Ratchell, or fragments of ftone.
Second, Limeftone, one foot thick, which contains no figured ftones.
Third, Sand.
Fourth, Argillaceous ftone.
Fifth, Bind.
Sixth, Coal.

Here it may be neceffary to obferve, that all beds of fand and gravel are adventitious affemblages of matter, and not original *ftrata*, whence it appears, that the above *ftratum* of limeftone is a recent production, formed fince the fea retired from that part of the earth, therefore not to be confideied as interfering with the general order of the *ftrata*.

The following obfervations feem to fhew, that gravel and fand are actually affemblages of adventitious matter.

A a 2   1. The

1. The river *Derwent* flows from the *gritftone ftratum*, and continues its courfe, ten or fifteen miles, at the foot of gritftone mountains ; throughout that fpace, the *bed* of the *river*, and its *adjacent meadows*, abound with *rounded gritftones* and *fand* which is manifeftly the granulated parts of the fame *ftratum*.

2. The river *Wee* continues its courfe many miles, through limeftone vallies, until it falls into the Derwent at Roufley : therefore the bed of that river, and its adjacent grounds, where flat, contain limeftones, chert, and other productions of the limeftone *ftrata*, rounded by attrition, and alfo granules of the fame *ftrata*.

Thus are the above rivers circumftanced down to to Roufley, where they unite. From thence to the river Trent, the bed of the Derwent, and its adjacent meadows, contain rounded grit, limeftone, and fand, as above.

Whence we may reafonably conclude, that all the above rounded ftones and beds of fand, have been actually depofited by the river Derwent, however diftant they may be found from its prefent courfe.

For inftance : wherever a pit is dug in the meadows between Derby and Chaddefden Hill, the gravel is compofed of fuch ftones and fand ; and yet the channel of the river has been confined to its prefent fituation
about

about two thoufand years: as appears by the remains of a bridge at Little-Chefter, faid to have
been conftructed by the Romans. This ancient
ruin is now immerfed a few feet in the river.

The fame kind of gravel as above, I faw dug up
at Ofmafton near the feat of Sir Robert Wilmot,
Baronet. The pit was about fix feet deep: and alfo
at Thurlftone, where the pit is now open for the repair
of public roads, and yet both the above places are
twenty or thirty feet above the level of the river
Derwent, and near one mile diftant.

Thefe inftances ferve to fhew, that the above beds
of gravel and fand are affemblages of adventitious
matter, and *not original ftrata*: Hence we may
conclude by analogy, that all beds of gravel where-
foever found, whether on mountains or in vallies,
have been depofited either by rivers or the action of
the fea, and that the ftones which compofe them
were rounded by attrition, as the ftones on a fea-
beach, or in rivers.

A little obfervation would furnifh innumerable inftances of the fame kind: I well remember feeing a
gravel pit about a mile fouth of Uppingham, containing rounded lime-ftones, fea-fhells, and a *ftratum*

tum of fand. The lime-ftone is fimilar to that of the Ketton-Quarry, which is peculiar for the figure of the granules which compofe it, being fpherical, and have the appearance of the roes of fifhes. The fand is manifeftly compofed of thofe granules, the grains being all of them fpherical. Now from the various circumftances attending this gravel-pit, as the rounded lime-ftones great and fmall; rounded fea-fhells, and fand; we cannot be a moment in doubt but this very pit muft have been originally a fea beach; and that the fand is the pulverized parts of that ftone.

Again. The counties of Chefter and Lancafter contain many beds of fand, which are occafionally dug up for the repair of roads and other purpofes. Thefe fand beds are frequently accompanied with a very curious phenomenon. At Maie, near the feat of Peter Brook, Efq. I faw a fand pit, containing the fragments of pit-coal and cinders depofited in a ftratified manner through a confiderable extent of the bank. I have alfo obferved the fame appearances at Mobberley near Knutsford, and in the road from Walton-bridge to Worfley in Lancafhire. In fhort, I fcarcely remember ever infpecting a bank of fand that was totally free from adventitious matter,

ter, or other evident marks of its having been depofited by the flowing of water. The above fragments of coal and cinders lay fix or feven feet below the furface of the earth.

Hence we may conclude that all beds of fand and gravel are affemblages of adventitious bodies and not original *ſtrata* : therefore wherever fand or gravel form the furface of the earth, they conceal the original *ſtrata* from our obfervation, and deprive us of the advantages of judging, whether coal or limeftone are contained in the lower regions of the earth, and more efpecially in flat countries where the *ſtrata* do not baffet.

In countries thus circumftanced, where coal or limeftone are wanted, it is advifable to make a few experiments by digging, or boreing through the gravel or fand to afcertain the qualities of the *ſtrata* underneath, whence we may infer with tolerable certainty what is contained below them.

It rarely happens that the argillaceous *ſtrata* are covered by gravel or fand ; but we have fome inftances of it, and therefore there may be many more.

At Nuttall near Nottingham, thofe beds of ftone or clay are covered by fand and gravel five or fix feet deep : therefore by viewing the furface not the leaft appearance of coal can be difcovered : this inftance alone may ferve to fhew the propriety of experimentally proving the lower *ftrata*.

What has been obferved concerning the origin of fand being the effects of attrition, is only to be underftood in a limited fenfe : for if we look upon an antient ftone edifice, it is eafy to obferve that the ftone is much impaired or wafted by the weather, and particularly on the South-fide, more than on the North, being more expofed to rain and wind than the other.

And it has already been obferved, that if we examine a ftone quarry we fhall find its upper furface decompofed as it were, by the operations of the weather, and reduced to grains of fand, which are continually wafhing down from the mountains and forming beds of fand in the vallies, rivers, and likewife in the fea.

Hence the origin of the gold-duft on the banks of the African rivers, and the irony fands on the American fhores.

Thus have the operations of the weather a conftant tendency to reftore the furface of the earth to its primative order and regularity. See Chap. VI.

Having

Having compleated my obfervations on the Derbyfhire *ftrata*, I purpofe giving fome account of an
extraordinary phenomenon which has frequently
happened in Haycliff and Ladywafh mines at
Eyam, and in Oden at Caftleton : the former are
thus circumftanced.

1. The minerals are contained in the fiffures of
the limeftone, N° 3. plate I. covered by a *ftratum*
of fhale and grit, which retain their full thicknefs of
fixty fathoms each.

2. The lead-ore and fpar contained in the above
mines are blended together fo as to produce the appearance of white Italian marble clouded with
black, and are fo extremely hard and compact as
to require blafting with-gun-powder, to feparate
them from the general mafs.

3. Thofe in the Ladywafh vein, are divided in
two equal parts parallel to the fides of the fiffure, as
reprefented by the line *a, a*, fig. 4. plate IX. They
may be compared to two flabs of marble, whofe
polifhed furfaces are abfolutely in contact with each
other without the leaft degree of cohefion.

4. Thefe naturally polifhed furfaces are not truly
flat, but in fome degree waved, as if fhot with a
carpenter's plane, confifting of various members.

B b   5. The

5. The two furfaces are coloured with lead ore, but as thinly laid as if only rubbed over with black-lead.

6. The vein in Haycliff Mine contains two of the above feams, and therefore may be compared to three flabs of marble, the middle one polifhed on both fides and in contact with the other two. The feparation of thefe flabs is reprefented by the two lines V, V, plate IX. fig. 5.

Thus are the above veins circumftanced : now what is yet more remarkable is this. If a fharp pointed pick is drawn down the vein with a fmall degree of force, the minerals begin to crackle, as fulphur excited to become electrical by rubbing; after this, in the fpace of two or three minutes, the folid mafs of the minerals explodes with much violence, and the fragments fly out, as if blafted with gun-powder.

Thefe effects have frequently happened, by which many workmen have been much wounded, but none killed, both in the Eyam mines and in that at Caftleton.

In the year 1738 a prodigious explofion happened in the mine called Haycliff.

The quantity of two hundred barrels of the above minerals were blown out at one blaft, each barrel,

I pre-

I prefume, contained no lefs than three or four hundred weight.

At the fame time a man was blown twelve fathoms perpendicular, and lodged upon a floor, or bunding, as the miners call it.

When the above explofion happened, the barrel, or tub, in which the minerals, &c. are raifed to the furface, happened to hang over the engine-fhaft, which is nearly feven feet wide, and five or fix hundred yards from the *forefield*, or *part*, where the explofion happened ; this barrel, though of confiderable weight, was lifted up in the hook on which it was fufpended ; and the people on the furface felt the ground fhake, as by an earthquake.

Such are the effects which have frequently been produced in all the above mines; but from what caufe they proceed I have not yet been able to difcover, nor even the leaft traces towards it.

When thefe wonderful effects firft happened they deterred the workmen for fome years from venturing to work the mines, but afterwards they availed themfelves of this extraordinary property. A man would go to the forefield, give a fcratch with his pick, and run away ; by which means he loofened as much of

B b 2 the

the minerals as could have been done by common workmanſhip with ten men in three months.

Theſe curious obſervations I received from Mr.
Mettam of Eyam, overſeer of the mines, who alſo ad-
dreſſed the following account of them to Mr. George
Tiſſington of Winſter.

" S I R,   *Eyam, 2 July*, 1768.

" I ſend you, by the bearer, two ſpecimens of our
" *ſlickenſides*,* containing all the variety of minerals
" where the exploſions happen ; they fly out in ſuch
" *ſlappits*,† ſmooth on one ſide.   The exploſions are
" ſometimes heard to the ſurface, and felt like an earth-
" quake ; they frequently blow out all the candles in
" the mine, and ſplit the *ſtemples* ‡ into ſplinters as
" ſmall as the twigs of a birch beeſom, to the diſtance
" of thirty or forty yards from the *forefield* § ; others
" are broke, and ſome of them become too ſhoit and
" drop out.

---

* *Slickenſides*, ſhining, as if poliſhed by art, on one ſide.
† *Slappits*, fragments of the minerals burſt out of the vein
‡ *Stemples*, joiſts laid acroſs fiſſures, when the minerals are cut out,
by way of making a floor, on which rubbiſh is depoſited, to ſave the
expence of raiſing it to the ſurface.
§ *Forefield*, that part of the vein under workmanſhip.

" The

" The fmooth fides lie face to face, and have the
" appearance of being fhot with a plane, confifting
" of various members. There is generally two of
" thefe divifions in our forefield at Haycliff, about
" eight or ten inches afunder, and a feam of white *keb-*
" *ble* ‖ in the middle of that fpace, half an inch thick,
" in which the miners rake down a fharp pointed
" pick until the crackling ceafeth ; then they run
" away, knowing that the explofion will follow in a
" minute or two. Sometimes a noife is heard like
" the beating of a church clock, after which the
" greateft explofions happen.

" I am yours, &c.

To Mr. George Tiffington,   Wᴵʟʟᴵᴀᴍ Mᴇᴛᴛᴀᴍ.
Winfter.

It was in the above mines that the workmen were
fo much alarmed on the firft of November 1755, about
ten o'clock in the morning, the time of the earthquake
fo fatal to Lifbon. The rocks which furrounded them,
were fo much difturbed, that foil, &c. fell from their
joints or fiffures ; and they likewife heard violent explofions, as it were of cannon. Being thus alarmed,

---

‖ *Kebble,* a white opaque fpar, calcarious, but not apt to break into rhomboidal forms

they

they left their subterraneous employment and fled to
the surface for safety. After some stay there and no
visible alterations ensuing, their fears began to abate,
when they ventured down again, and to their great
surprize found nothing material had happened in
their absence. I have related these particulars, as
small circumstances sometimes throw considerable
lights on physical researches.

Here it is necessary to remark that the preceding
observations on the Derbyshire *strata* leave much
room to wish for further information; they may
however help to point out the road to a careful ob-
server, and serve to excite philosophers to exert
themselves in researches of so much importance.

T H E

THE

CONCLUSION.

LET us now take a view of the preceding inquiries.

The globe, which we now inhabit, was originally a chaotic, heterogeneous mafs, and progreffively formed into an habitable world.

By the union of fimilar particles, air was freed fiom the general mafs, and formed a muddy, impure atmofphere. Water, being next in levity, fucceeded the air, and furrounded the earth with an univerfal fea. In procefs of time, thefe two elements became fre·d from grofs matter, and fit for animal life.

The marine inhabitants were then created, and replenifhed the ocean from pole to pole.

The moon being coeval with the earth, was inftrumental in the production of iflands, by means of the tides, and divided the waters which prevailed over the earth.

Iflands

Iflands being thus formed by the tides, many of the marine inhabitants were buried in the mud; and this mud, in procefs of time concreting into ftone, the animals perifhed, and their *exuviæ* became a ftony fubftance.

The *ftrata* were alfo formed by the union of fimilar particles, and therefore obtained an uniform *concentric* arrangement, furrounding the center of the earth, as fo many fhells may be fuppofed to furround an egg; and in this uniform ftate became ftone, and acquired the greateft degree of cohefion and firmnefs.

Subterraneous fire being now univerfally generated in the fame *ftratum* or central part of the earth, by its expanfive force gradually diftended their incumbent *ftrata*, like a bladder forceably blown, and, by elevating the bottom of the ocean more than the primitive iflands, deluged the whole earth. Subterraneous fire ftill increafing, its expanfive force gradually burft the incumbent *ftrata*, and opened their fiffures more and more, until the two oceans of melted matter and water came into contact, whence a violent explofion enfued, which tore the globe into millions of fragments, and threw them into every poffible degree of confufion, fome of them being more elevated, and others more depreffed. Hence

arofe

arofe an infinite number of fubterraneous caverns, apparently many miles, or many hundreds of miles, below the bottom of the primitive ocean. Into thefe caverns the waters defcended, and left the mountains and continents naked and expofed, which had no exiftence prior to that æra.*

The great increafe of terreftrial furface, and contraction of the fea, was productive of an equal change in the temperature of the air and feafons of the year; (See chap. xiii) for by means of this alteration, commenced the burning heats in fummer and the feverities of winter ; and deftroyed that univerfal equality in the feafons which prevailed over the earth in the firft ages, (See chap. xiv.) when fpring and autumn reigned together, and trees were conftantly loaded with bloffoms and fruit.

Thus were the calls of human nature fatisfied without art or labour ; neither were there any ftorms or tempefts, jealoufies or fears, amongft men, to invade their repofe ; but they flept in perfect fecurity on the ever verdant turf. Our firft parents being thus plentifully provided with food, and a climate which required no

* See chap. xii.

C c

protection

protection from the inclemency of the weather; 'tis no wonder they lived together in perfect harmony, without law, as the ancients have afferted.

But no fooner did mountains and continents emerge from beneath the deep, than the year became divided into fummer and winter, fpring and autumn. From that æra, the products of the earth were only obtained by *art* and *labour*. It then became neceffary for men to *fow* and *cultivate* the *earth* : alfo to lay up for winter's ftore, and to protect themfelves from the inclemency of the feafons. Thus commenced *property* ; for he that fowed, would expect to *reap* the *fruits* of his labour : and *he* who *built* an *houfe*, would expect to enjoy it.

NECESSITY, therefore, gave birth to *property*, and deftroyed that equality and harmony which univerfally prevailed amongft mankind in the firft ages of the world : for experience fhews, that men who are born in rude and favage climates are naturally of a ferocious difpofition ; and that a fertile foil, which leaves nothing to wifh for, foftens their manners and inclines them to humanity.

Such, however, is apparently the refult of the preceding chapters. Should the obfervations I have made,

or

or the inferences I have drawn, prove inftrumental in throwing any light on ancient hiftory, *facred* or *profane*; or of leading to the difcovery of thofe things which have a tendency to promote the welfare of mankind; I fhall not think my time has been fpent in vain.

THE END.

POST-

POSTSCRIPT.

GYPSUM, having escaped my notice in the Appendix, renders the following observations necessary; since it is the production of a Derbyshire *stratum*.

GYPSUM is usually called *alabaster*, or *plaister*. Its uses for chimney-pieces, monuments, floors, &c. &c. are well known.

It has very different modifications in the earth, being found in large nodulous masses, and stratified. The latter is fibrous; and its fibers run nearly at right angles from its upper or lower surface. It is of an opaque white, and uniform in its colour. The former is neither fibrous nor laminated, but composed of granules, as sugar, and breaks alike in all directions. Some of these masses are of a fine opaque white, like statuary marble; others are variegated with different colours, as red, green, and blueish; these colours are sometimes so blended with the gypseous matter, as to produce the appearance of Italian marble clouded with blackish veins. It takes a good polish, and though not so hard as marble, it is deservedly esteemed for various internal ornamental purposes in architecture, &c. but will not indure the weather.

To

To the above we may add the laminated *gypsum*, which is generally dug up at various depths, from 10 to 100 yards. Though I have not seen the particular parts whence this plated *gypsum* is taken, yet it has the appearance of being stratified, and is generally as transparent as the finest colourless crystal.

All the above *gypsums* are found in *marl*, or calcarious earth; both in Derbyshire, Nottinghamshire, Staffordshire, and Cheshire. The nodulous masses are dug up at Chelaston, &c. near Derby; and also near Sudbury, in Staffordshire; and at several places in the south part of Nottinghamshire: and also the fibrous kind, which may be conveniently observed at Clifton, the seat of Sir Gervas Clifton, Bart. near Nottingham, by the river Trent.

The plated *gypsum* is generally dug up in Cheshire, where pits are sunk for salt springs and salt rock.

Selenites, though a gypseous body, is only found in clay which is not calcarious, but contains a vitriolic acid; it is laminated, transparent, and assumes a particular mode of crystallization, well known to naturalists.

It may be necessary further to observe, that *gypsum* appears to be as much a production of marl, or calcarious earth, as flint is of chalk, or chert of limestone.

Chert

Chert is a production of the limeftone *ftrata* in Derbyfhire. It is a flinty fubftance, in nodulous forms, as flint in chalk, though fometimes a little ftratified. Some of it plentifully abounds with the impreffions of *entrochi*, which have manifeftly been inclofed in the folid fubftance of the *chert*, though not the leaft fragment of them is now remaining. Its colour is fimilar to that of other flints; but when ftratified, is generally a good black. It is fometimes fo like in colour to the limeftone in which it is inclofed, as to be only diftinguifhed by its not effervefcing with acids.

Chert may be conveniently obferved in the cliffs at Cromford, &c. &c.

The *ftratum* of marl containing *gypfum*, is very thick. I have known pits funk into it eighty or an hundred yards deep, and never heard of its being cut through: nor do I remember ever feeing any other than adventitious matter incumbent on it.

Marl is fometimes much indurated, and even concreted to a perfect limeftone. I have feen fome inftances of its being burnt to lime, but thefe are not commonly obferved.   2

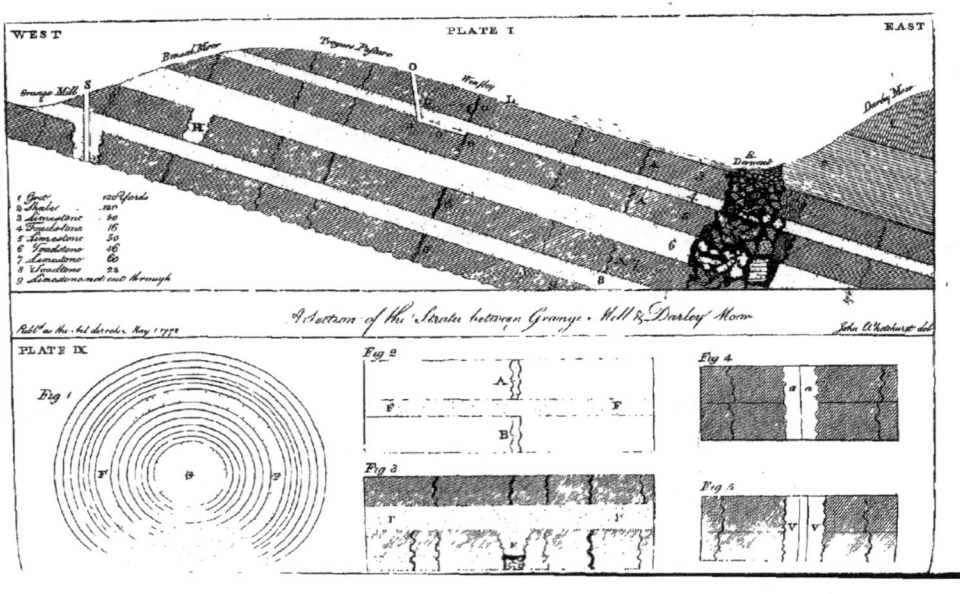

A Section of the Strata between Grange Mill & Darley Moor

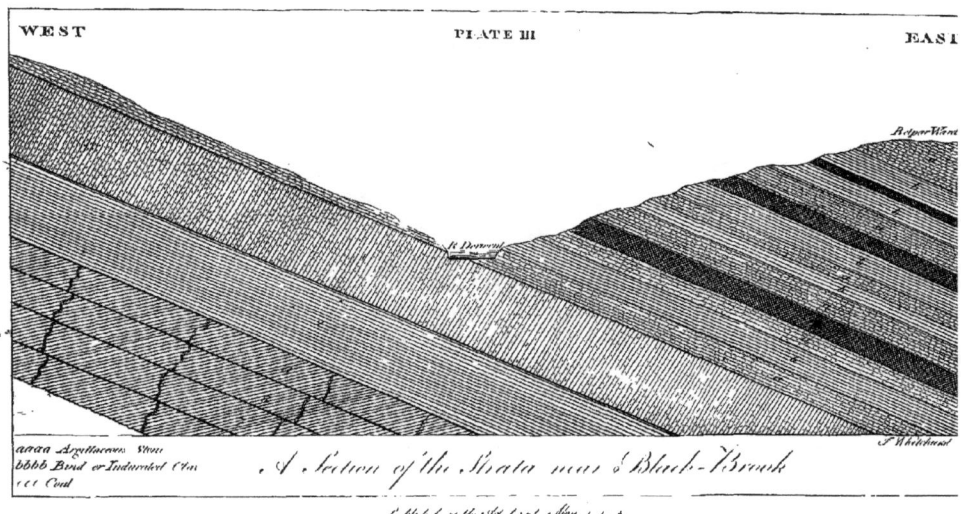

Redyer-Went

R. Derwent

J. Whitehurst

aaaa Argillaceous Stone
bbbb Bind or Indurated Clay
cc Coal

A Section of the Strata near Black-Brook

Published as the Act directs May 1778.

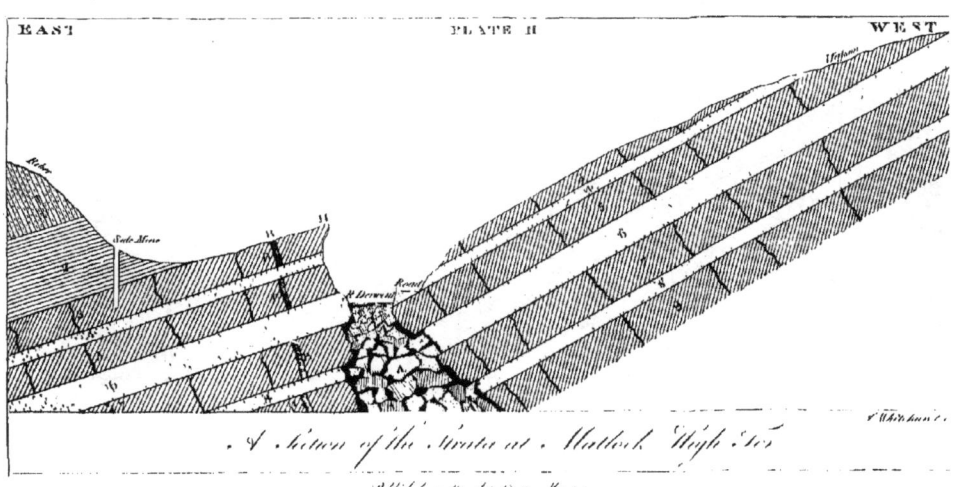

Upland

Rider

Sale Mine

R. Derwent

Road

J. Whitehurst

A Section of the Strata at Matlock High Tor

Published as the Act directs May 1778.

PLATE V

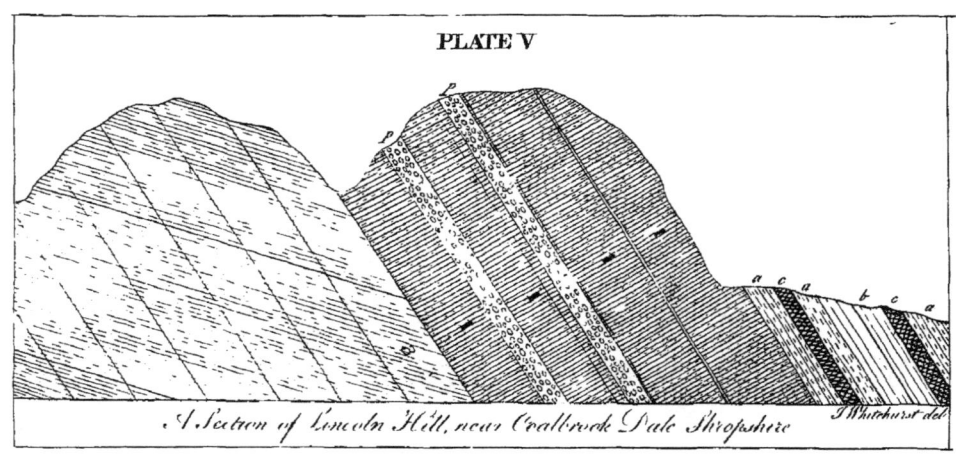

A Section of Lincoln Hill, near Coalbrook Dale Shropshire

J Whitehurst del.

WEST   PLATE

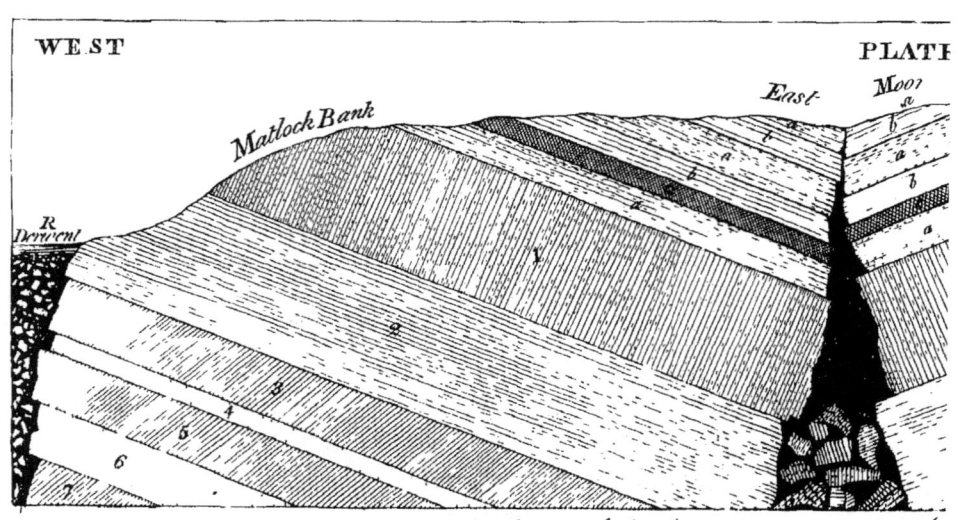

A Section of the Strata between the River

Published as the Act directs May

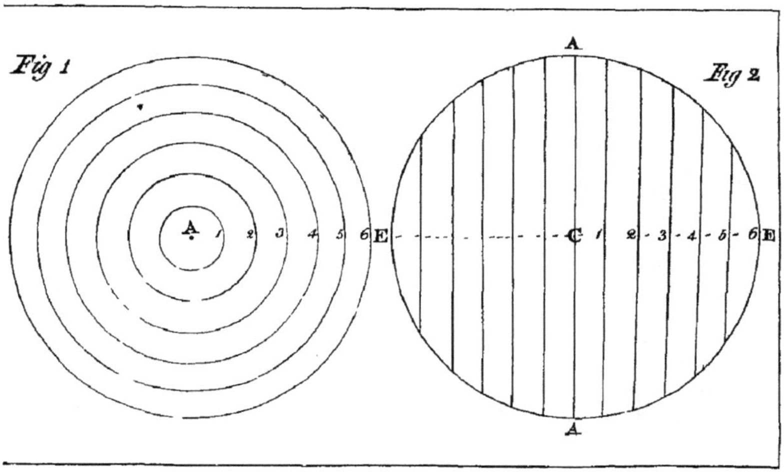

Fig 1

Fig 2

A · 1 2 3 4 5 6 E

A — C 1 · 2 · 3 · 4 · 5 · 6 E

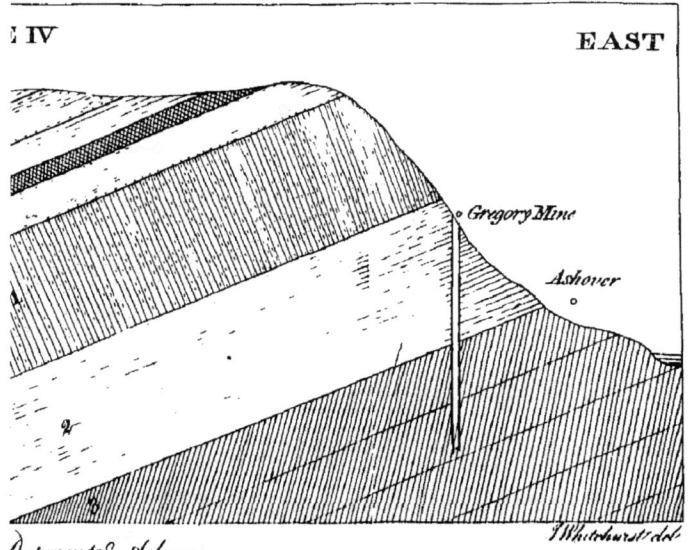

IV

EAST

∘ Gregory Mine

Ashover ∘

Derwent & Ashover
778

J. Whitehurst del.

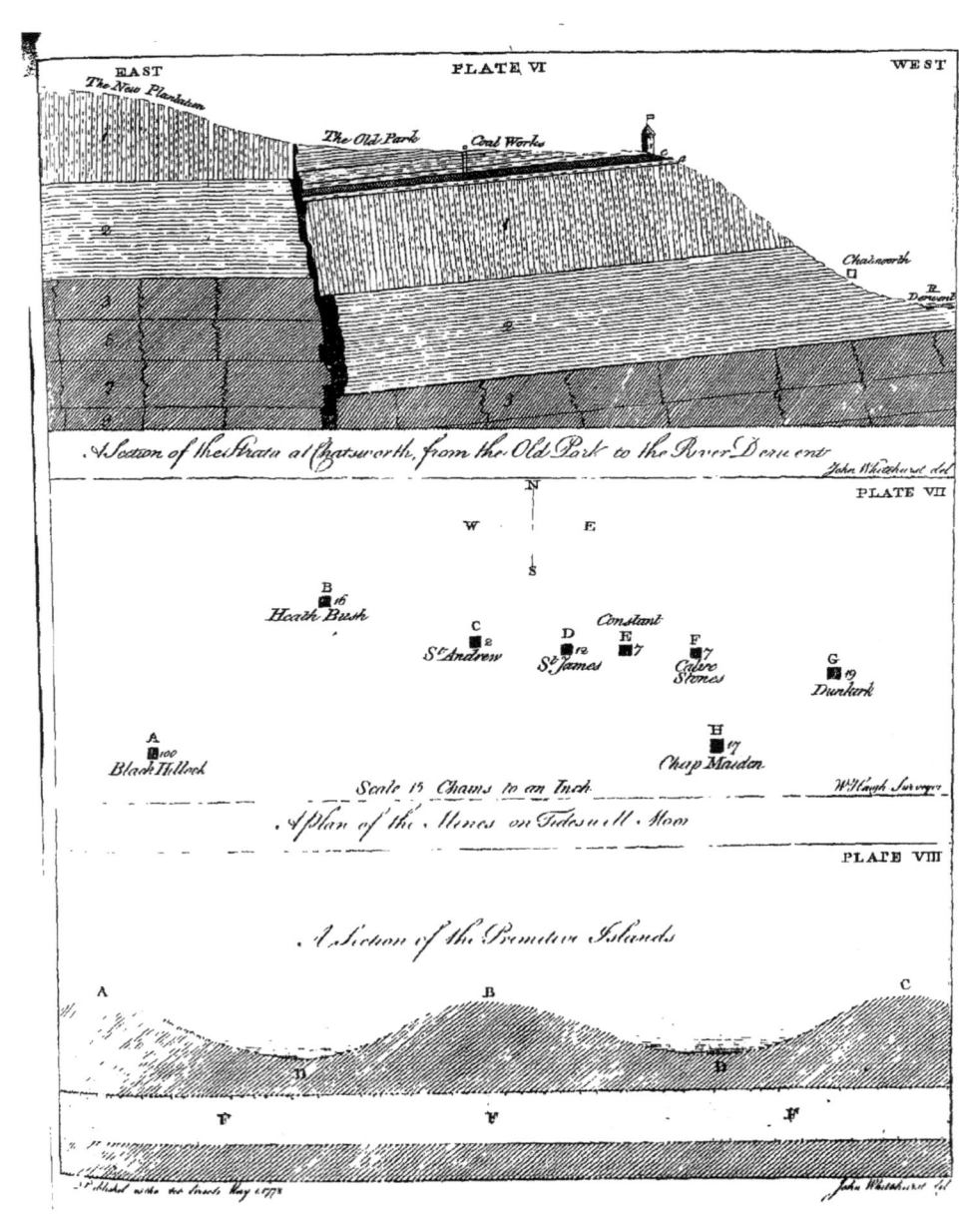

EAST   PLATE VI   WEST

The New Plantation

The Old Park   Coal Works

Chatsworth

R. Derwent

A Section of the Strata at Chatsworth, from the Old Park to the River Derwent.

John Whitehurst del.

PLATE VII

N

W   E

S

B 16
Heath Bush

C 2
St Andrew

D 12
St James

Constant

E 7

F 7
Calvre Stones

G 19
Dunkirk

A 100
Black Hillock

H 17
Chap Maiden

Scale 13 Chains to an Inch.

W. Haugh Surveyor

A Plan of the Mines on Tideswell Moor

PLATE VIII

A Section of the Primitive Islands

A   B   C

D   D

F   F   F

Published as the Act directs May 1. 1778

John Whitehurst del.

Lightning Source UK Ltd.
Milton Keynes UK
UKHW051427031022
409740UK00014B/77